Collaborative Practice in
Critical Care S

This practical and evidence-based workbook offers a series of assessment, implementation and evaluation activities for professionals working in critical care contexts. Designed to improve the quality of care delivery, it looks both at collaboration between professionals and between patients and/or family members.

Collaborative Practice in Critical Care Settings:

- identifies the issues relating to the "current state" of collaboration in critical care through a series of assessment activities;
- provides a series of interventional activities which can address shortfalls of collaboration previously identified; and
- offers advice on generating evidence for the effects of any interventions implemented.

The activities presented in this book are based on extensive empirical research, ensuring this book takes into account the everyday work environment of professionals in critical care units. It is suitable for practitioners and educators, as well as patient safety leads and managers.

Scott Reeves is professor in Interprofessional Research at the Faculty of Health, Social Care and Education, Kingston and St George's, University of London, UK, and Editor-in-Chief of the *Journal of Interprofessional Care*.

Janet Alexanian is a senior research associate at St Michael's Hospital, Toronto, Canada. She received her doctorate in anthropology at the University of California, Irvine, in 2009.

Deborah Kendall-Gallagher is an adjunct assistant professor at the University of Texas Health Science Center, San Antonio School of Nursing, USA.

Todd Dorman is a critical care physician. He is the Senior Associate Dean for Education Coordination and the Associate Dean for Continuing Medical Education for the Johns Hopkins School of Medicine, USA.

Simon Kitto is a professor in the Department of Innovation in Medical Education and Director of Research in the Office of Continuing Professional Development at the University of Ottawa, Canada.

CAIPE Collaborative Practice series

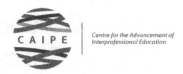

Founded in 1987, CAIPE is a charity and company limited by guarantee which promotes and develops interprofessional education with and through its members.

It works with like-minded organisations in the UK and overseas to improve collaborative practice, patient safety and quality of care by professions learning and working together. CAIPE's contributions to IPE include publications, development workshops, consultancy, commissioned studies and international partnerships, projects and networks.

CAIPE not only offers expertise and experience, but also provides an independent perspective which can facilitate collaboration across the boundaries between education and health, health and social care, and beyond.

Membership of CAIPE is open to individuals, students and organisations such as academic institutions, independent and public service providers in the UK and overseas.

For further information about CAIPE and other benefits of membership go to www.caipe.org.uk.

Collaborative Practice in Critical Care Settings

A Workbook

Scott Reeves,
Janet Alexanian,
Deborah Kendall-Gallagher,
Todd Dorman
and Simon Kitto

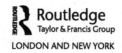

Routledge
Taylor & Francis Group

LONDON AND NEW YORK

First published 2019
by Routledge
2 Park Square, Milton Park, Abingdon, Oxon OX14 4RN

and by Routledge
711 Third Avenue, New York, NY 10017

Routledge is an imprint of the Taylor & Francis Group, an informa business

© 2019 Scott Reeves, Janet Alexanian, Deborah Kendall-Gallagher,
Todd Dorman, and Simon Kitto

The right of Scott Reeves, Janet Alexanian, Deborah Kendall-Gallagher,
Todd Dorman, and Simon Kitto to be identified as authors of this work has
been asserted by them in accordance with sections 77 and 78 of the
Copyright, Designs and Patents Act 1988.

British Library Cataloguing-in-Publication Data
A catalogue record for this book is available from the British Library

Library of Congress Cataloging-in-Publication Data
Names: Reeves, Scott, 1967- author. | Alexanian, Janet, author. |
Kendall-Gallagher, Deborah, author. | Dorman, Todd, author. | Kitto, Simon
(Sociologist), author.
Title: Collaborative practice in critical care settings : a workbook / Scott Reeves,
Janet Alexanian, Deborah Kendall-Gallagher, Todd Dorman and Simon Kitto.
Description: Abingdon, Oxon ; New York, NY : Routledge, 2019. | Includes
bibliographical references and index.
Identifiers: LCCN 2018019316| ISBN 9781138633483 (hardback) | ISBN
9781138633490 (pbk.) | ISBN 9781315207308 (ebook)
Subjects: | MESH: Critical Care—organization & administration | Intensive
Care Units—organization & administration | Intersectoral Collaboration |
Professional-Patient Relations | Evidence-Based Practice
Classification: LCC RA975.5.I56 | NLM WX 218 | DDC 362.17/4068—dc23
LC record available at https://lccn.loc.gov/2018019316

ISBN: 978-1-138-63348-3 (hbk)
ISBN: 978-1-138-63349-0 (pbk)
ISBN: 978-1-315-20730-8 (ebk)

Typeset in Sabon and Helvetica Neue
by Florence Production Ltd, Stoodleigh, Devon, UK

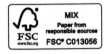

Printed and bound in Great Britain by
TJ International Ltd, Padstow, Cornwall

Contents

About the authors

Scott Reeves is a social scientist who has been undertaking health professions education and health services research for over twenty years. His main interests are focused on developing conceptual, empirical and theoretical knowledge to inform the design and implementation of interprofessional education and practice activities. He has received millions of dollars in grants from a range of funding bodies across the world and published hundreds of peer-reviewed papers, book chapters, textbooks, editorials and monographs. He is currently Professor in Interprofessional Research at the Faculty of Health, Social Care and Education, Kingston and St George's, University of London, UK, as well as Editor-in-Chief of the *Journal of Interprofessional Care*. After spending a decade in London at City University he moved to North America, initially to Canada where he was the inaugural Director of Research, Centre for Faculty Development, St Michael's Hospital and Professor in the Faculty of Medicine at the University of Toronto. Moving then to the USA, he was appointed as the Founding Director, of the Center for Innovation in Interprofessional Education as well as Professor in the Department of Social and Behavioral Sciences and Department of Medicine, University of California, San Francisco. He holds a number of visiting academic positions in a variety of countries, including, Japan, Ireland, New Zealand, USA, Canada, UK and Sweden.

Janet Alexanian is a senior researcher at St Michael's Hospital in Toronto. She completed her doctorate in anthropology at the University of California, Irvine, in 2009. She was the lead researcher for multi-sited ethnographic study examining interprofessional collaboration and patient and family involvement in the delivery of care in eight intensive care units in the USA and Canada, as well as a CIHR-funded implementation trial of a family involvement tool. Janet has worked as an adjunct professor in the Departments of Anthropology at California State University, Fullerton, Dominguez Hills, and the University of California, Irvine.

Deborah Kendall-Gallagher is an adjunct assistant professor at the University of Texas Health Science Center, San Antonio School of Nursing, USA. She teaches doctoral nursing students about system transformation with an emphasis on the role of leadership in building interprofessional teams to influence quality, patient safety, and health policy. She has over twenty years of experience working with clinicians and organisations to improve patient safety and quality across the continuum of care; her research focuses on interprofessional education and practice.

Todd Dorman is a critical care physician. He is the Senior Associate Dean for Education Coordination and the Associate Dean for Continuing Medical Education for the Johns Hopkins School of Medicine, USA. He is a Professor and Vice Chair for Critical Care in the Department of Anesthesiology and Critical Care Medicine and has joint appointments as a Professor in Internal Medicine, Surgery and The School of Nursing. Previously he served as the Director of the Multidisciplinary Critical Care Fellowship Program, Director of the Division of Adult Critical Care Medicine, Co-Director of the Surgical Intensive Care Units, Medical Director of the Adult Post-anesthesiology Care Units and Medical Director of Respiratory Care Services. He co-chairs the committee on interactions with industry and serves on the conflict of commitment committee. He also co-chairs the departmental associate professor mentorship committee.

Simon Kitto is a medical sociologist who has been working in health professions education research since 2002. He is a professor in the Department of Innovation in Medical Education and Director of Research in the Office of Continuing Professional Development at the University of Ottawa, Canada. He is also Editor-in-Chief of the *Journal of Continuing Education in the Health Professions*. His main research interests are studying how structural, historical and socio-cultural variables shape interprofessional clinical practice, educational settings and activities. His current research focuses on the nature and role of continuing interprofessional education and practice within the nexus of patient safety, quality improvement and implementation science intervention design and practice.

Scott Reeves

Scott died suddenly soon after completing this workbook. The last of his many interprofessional publications, it exemplifies his achievements as the outstanding interprofessional scholar of his generation bringing out the best in those of us who were privileged to work with him. Tributes to Scott from around the world can be found on www.caipe.org/.

Hugh Barr
President, CAIPE
May 2018

Acknowledgements

We would like to thank our editors, Hugh Barr and Alison Machin, for their guidance and critical feedback during the writing of this book.

Scott would like to also acknowledge the support of his family, Ruth, William, Ewan and Joshua, who provided much needed encouragement.

Introduction

....

This workbook's aim is to offer readers a series of assessment, implementation and evaluation activities designed to improve collaboration (interprofessionally and also between providers and patients/family members) in critical care contexts in order to improve the quality and safety of care delivery. Throughout the chapters, the workbook focuses on three interlocking elements:

- how to identify the issues related to collaboration in critical care settings through a series of assessment activities;
- how to develop a series of interventional activities which can begin to address the identified shortfalls in collaboration, and;
- how to generate evaluative evidence to help measure the effects of any interventions implemented.

As such, the chapters in the book provide descriptions of a variety of different activities all designed to enhance collaborative practice between critical care staff (i.e. professionals, managers, support workers) and also enhance collaboration between staff and patients' family members. The book also offers a series of appendices which contain a variety of materials aimed to support the facilitation of the collaborative activities which are described in the chapters.

Materials for this workbook are based on an unpublished toolkit which was generated from a two-year, multi-sited ethnographic study of eight intensive care units (ICU) across North America. The actual study involved gathering over 1,000 hours of observation of interprofessional work in ICUs providing services to adults, as well as interactions between healthcare providers and patient/family members. In addition, the study conducted numerous clinician interviews (e.g. physicians, nurses, pharmacists) and family member interviews. As a result, the study has generated a rich and unique empirical insight into the everyday work of professionals in the intensive care settings (see Appendix 1 for more details on this study).

While the materials for the book were generated in a North American context, the ideas, activities and approaches offered here have, arguably, a much broader resonance for readers based across the globe given the similarities related to collaboration we have found both in our professional experiences and in the literature.

OUR FOCUS

This workbook focuses on collaboration in critical care settings across a range of different national contexts. As authors, we have personal/professional experience of collaboration in critical care from four different countries – Australia, Canada, the UK and USA. Our professional/academic networks expand this reach into other countries, including, Brazil, Denmark, Germany, Japan, South Africa, Sweden and Switzerland.

While we have a specific focus on collaboration in critical care, our focus is nevertheless inclusive in terms of the different individuals who occupy this setting. We therefore draw on experiences from medicine, nursing, respiratory therapy, pharmacy and social work, but also draw upon the perspectives of administrators, support staff, as well as patients and their family members.

Overall, the focus of this workbook is to enrich readers understanding of key issues linked to collaboration in critical care settings – related to collaboration between staff and collaboration between patients/families and staff. It also aims to provide a set of ideas, activities and approaches aimed at promoting these differing forms of collaboration in relation to their design, implementation and evaluation.

WHY READ THIS WORKBOOK?

This workbook is addressed to people (providers, family members, managers, policy makers, researchers, educators and students) who are based in critical care settings – providing care, managing, engaged in teaching/learning, involved in policy making – or those who have an interest in understanding more about the nature of collaboration in this context.

The book aims to provide text that offers a range of key insights, ideas and activities regarding collaboration in critical care, specifically related to identifying factors that affect collaboration as well as suggestions to how to intervene to improve identified problems and how to develop evidence to understand the effects of any interventions. Our overall intention is to provide readers with a thoughtful yet critical account of different forms of collaboration in critical care and how it is possible to enhance any deficiencies to help improve the quality and safety of the care delivered in this setting.

The book employs an evidence-based approach which has been carefully analysed and synthesised to generate a wide range of practical ideas and approaches that offer advice to help inform critical care providers, family members, managers, policy makers, researchers, educators and students.

The book aims to provide evidence and guidance for those who wish to commission, design, develop, and implement interventions to improve critical care collaboration as well as evaluate the effects of these interventions in robust manner.

Finally, this book contains a set of appendices which contain further supporting information aimed to enhance the facilitation of the collaborative interventions identified in the chapters.

OUR FRAMEWORK

Throughout this workbook we draw on the PROC framework (Figure 0.1) developed to help understand the nature of interprofessional teamwork (Reeves et al. 2010). As indicated in this figure, the PROC framework consists of the following four domains:

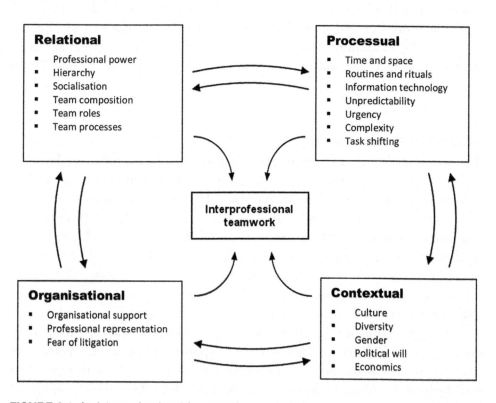

FIGURE 0.1 An interprofessional framework

- Relational – factors which directly affect the relationships shared by professions such as professional power and socialisation.
- Processual – factors such as space and time which affect how the work of the team is carried out across different workplace situations.
- Organisational – factors that affect the local organisational environment in which the interprofessional team operates.
- Contextual – factors related to the broader social, political and economic landscape in which the team is located.

As the arrows in Figure 0.1 suggest, each of these factors are linked with one domain and have the ability to affect interprofessional teamwork in different ways.

For simplicity the PROC framework has been arranged using four domains. However, it should be noted that these domains and their embedded factors are not mutually exclusive, so there is some inter-connection between them. For example, while the factor "professional power" has been included in the relational domain, its effects will also be felt in the processual and organisational domains. Similarly, while "culture" is located in the contextual domain, its influence will also span relational and processual domains.

For a more detailed explanation of the PROC framework see Reeves et al. (2010). In addition, for information on how the framework has been implemented in other studies, see Mischo-Kelling et al. (2015) and Pinho et al. (2018).

HOW TO USE THIS WORKBOOK
The ideas, activities and tools presented in this workbook can be used collectively, as stand-alone activities, or can be incorporated into an existing interprofessional team activity such as the CUSP (Comprehensive Unit Based Safety Program – see Appendix 2). The activities and tools can be employed individually, consecutively, or simultaneously. While it is advisable to have a staff member or an external resource dedicated to serving as facilitator for the quality improvement process, this is not necessary. The workbook is designed to be used by those based in critical care settings who are interested in enhancing interprofessional collaboration and/or family member involvement.

Although in practical terms it will usually be local hospital patient safety committees or CUSP safety teams whose support will be needed before the activities in this workbook can be implemented. Indeed, it is important to initially have this level of support as patient safety leads from these committees or teams will in turn need to liaise with hospital management to ensure that the toolkit has wider organisational "buy in". Once the local patient safety committees/teams are involved, discussion can be undertaken in terms of planning the roll out (implementation) of the different tools.

THE IMPORTANCE OF CONTEXT

It is important to consider the nature of local context (i.e. hospital and unit level) when examining teamwork, collaboration, reporting and error. By considering these concepts within their context we can understand the deeper meanings, and can then tailor interventions to improve patient safety within that specific context. The extensive research and holistic conceptual framework informing this workbook make it clear that patient safety initiatives need to consider how professionals perceive errors, as well as unpack the assumptions surrounding collaboration in critical care settings. It can also be difficult to foster collaborative relationships with patients and families when there is conceptual ambiguity around what patient and family involvement is.

OVERVIEW

This workbook is divided into the following chapters, which aim to take the reader across a range of interprofessional collaboration/teamwork and patient/family member involvement issues which affect critical care settings.

Chapter 1 sets the scene for the workbook by providing a selected review of the interprofessional and patient/family literature related to critical care settings, and covers a range of issues such as building infrastructure, paying attention to local context, and giving patients and their families voice.

Chapter 2 offers a series of activities designed to assess the nature of interprofessional collaboration a critical care setting and also intervene to enhance its quality. The chapter also outlines some ideas for evaluation of these activities.

Chapter 3 presents a series of activities to allow critical care staff to reflect upon their own understanding about patient/family involvement. The chapter also offers a range of suggestions to evaluate these activities.

Chapter 4 describes an activity designed for critical care staff to collaboratively identify issues that affect interprofessional collaboration and patient/family member involvement. It also provides a series of interprofessional interventions which aim to improve the identified issues from the activity.

Chapter 5 provides guidance on how to design and implement robust evidence to understand the effects of the activities and interventions described in the previous three chapters.

Chapter 6 presents key conclusions based on the activities presented in the previous chapters, to enhance collaboration amongst professionals and between patients and families based in critical care settings.

Appendices – a series of twelve appendices are also offered which provide additional information and resources for the materials presented in the chapters.

CHAPTER 1

Examining effective collaboration in critical care settings

························

INTRODUCTION

In this chapter we provide an overview of the literature related to effective collaboration among critical care professionals and between patient/family members. Following an extensive literature search we found that four central themes were key to developing and sustaining these differing forms of collaboration.

BACKGROUND

Interprofessional collaboration provides the foundation for delivering safe, efficient, patient-centred care. Effective collaborative practice engages different healthcare providers, patients and their family members. Collaborative practice is seen as a key mechanism for achieving the end goal of improving patient outcomes (Lutfiyya et al. 2016a). However, limited teamwork, poor coordination and ineffectual communication are regularly cited as precursors to preventable healthcare-related adverse outcomes (e.g. Reeves et al. 2017a). In addition to harm caused to patients, adverse events are expensive. Van Den Bos et al. (2011), for instance, estimated that in the USA in 2008, the annual cost of measurable clinical error resulting in harm was $17.1 billion.

Effective interprofessional collaboration is essential in critical care settings due to the clinical vulnerability of the patient population, many of whom may not be able to give voice to their concerns (e.g. Happ, 2000), and the complexity of technology in these environments. According to Dietz et al. (2014), the combination of clinical vulnerability and technological complexity means that "the margin of error is thin, and the consequences of errors are profound" (p. 912).

Critical care patients' lives depend on the ability of their healthcare providers to problem-solve quickly, collaboratively and effectively to give them the best outcome possible (Kendall-Gallagher et al. 2016; Manthous et al. 2011). Learning to function effectively together as a team in critical care is a skill developed over time through evidence-informed, mentored practice (Manthous et al. 2011). A growing body of evidence suggests a multitude of interrelated factors influence the quality of effective interprofessional collaboration (Courtenay et al. 2013; Dietz et al. 2014; Manthous et al. 2011; Paradis et al. 2014; Reeves et al. 2015a; 2017a).

Family members are increasingly being recognised as having an important role on the critical care healthcare team (Davidson et al. 2017; Olding et al. 2016). Greater engagement of patients' family members during a critical care admission benefits both patient and family – reported benefits include a decrease in family member psychological stress associated with their loved one's critical care stay and an increase in family members' effectiveness when caring for the patient (e.g. Gerritsen et al. 2017).

KEY THEMES FROM THE LITERATURE
As noted above, our review of the literature revealed the following four key themes related to collaboration within a critical care context:

- building the infrastructure to support sustainable improvement;
- understanding how local context impacts collaboration;
- creating psychologically safe environments;
- giving patients and their families a voice.

Below we describe and discuss each of these areas to help provide an insight into some of the issues affecting collaboration between critical care professionals, patients and their families.

BUILDING THE INFRASTRUCTURE TO SUPPORT SUSTAINABLE IMPROVEMENT
Critical care units vary considerably in size, structure, model of care, outcomes, and cost (Fanelli & Zangrandi, 2017; Prin & Wunsch, 2012; Vincent et al. 2014). In the United States, for example, the annual cost of critical care has been estimated to be in the range of $80 billion (Halpern & Pastores, 2015; Kahn & Rubenfeld, 2015). Numerous strategies have been introduced to improve patient outcomes and reduce costs including use of intensivists (Valentin et al. 2011; Weled et al. 2015), evidence-based protocols (Pronovost

et al. 2010), and interprofessional daily rounds (Kim et al. 2010). However, use of these strategies, either individually or collectively, has produced mixed improvements in quality (Dixon-Woods et al. 2013; Kerlin et al. 2017).

Quantitative research findings suggest interprofessional collaborative models of care may be an effective framework for achieving overall improvement in critical care outcomes (Checkly et al. 2014). For example, Kim et al. (2010) used multivariate logistic regression to determine if interprofessional care teams had an independent effect on 30-day mortality in a risk-adjusted sample of 107, 324 adult ICU patients across 112 hospitals by linking patient-level discharge data with data from a multi-centre, hospital-level organisational survey. The independent variable was the presence or absence of interprofessional rounds (Kim et al. p. 370). These authors found that the odds of death were significantly lower with use of interprofessional teams, noting that "survival benefit of intensivist physician staffing is in part explained by the presence of multidisciplinary teams in high-intensity staffed ICUs" (Kim et al. p. 369). In contrast, a study by Costa et al. (2015) involving forty-nine ICUs across twenty-five hospitals which aimed to explore the impact of daytime intensivist physician staffing on risk-adjusted ICU adult patient in-hospital mortality. Controlling for interprofessional rounds and clinical protocols, the authors found no significant association between daytime intensivists and reduced odds of mortality. More recently, the American Thoracic Society published a systematic review (eighteen studies) and meta-analysis (four studies) examining adjusted effects of night-time intensivists on adult ICU patient mortality and ICU length of stay (Kerlin et al. 2017). The authors found that night-time intensivist staffing was not significantly associated with either mortality (odds ratio, 0.99; 95% confidence interval, 0.75–1.29) or patient length of stay and concluded that other types of ICU staffing models such as "interprofessional care delivery models" may need to be considered as a pathway for improving ICU outcomes (Kerlin et al. p. 390).

Qualitative studies exploring interprofessional collaboration teamwork across critical care settings provide a window for understanding why efforts to improve critical care outcomes through introduction of quality improvement (QI) interventions, such as clinical protocols and presence of intensivists, produce inconsistent results (Dixon-Woods et al. 2013; Reeves et al. 2017b). In particular, a growing body of qualitative data suggests that failure to understand the underlying "social processes and mechanisms that produced the outcomes" impedes meaningful and sustainable improvements in quality (Dixon-Woods et al. 2011, p. 168). For example, Costa and colleagues (2014) interviewed sixty-four ICU clinicians composed of clinical pharmacists, dieticians, nurses, nurse managers, physicians and respiratory therapists across seven ICUs to identify factors that facilitated their collaborative efforts. Two types of facilitating factors emerged from the data – cultural and structural – with each factor working independently, as well as interdependently, to facilitate interprofessional collaboration. Structural factors were seen as tools that improved the efficiency and effectiveness of communication among ICU clinicians such as checklists, clinical protocols and daily rounds; whereas cultural factors addressed modifiable, non-technical factors related to team member accessibility, trust, value and leadership (Costa et al. 2014).

As a number of studies have indicated, building an effective interprofessional team within critical care requires forethought regarding fostering positive interactions that create an environment of trust, respect, and psychological safety (e.g. Manthous & Hollingshead, 2011; Paradis et al. 2014; Reeves et al. 2015a). However, as Manthous & Hollingshead, (2011) note, a "team approach [. . .] does not arise by accident or spontaneous generation but rather through cultivation of principles and practices rooted in the social and behavioural sciences" (p.17). In addition, effective leadership across the team is also required (Caldwell et al. 2008).

Importantly, findings from recent reviews examining interprofessional teamwork and collaboration have indicated that failure to address the underlying social context of care that drives clinician, managerial and organisational behaviours is one of the most significant impediments to achieving meaningful and sustainable improvements in quality and safety (Dixon-Woods et al. 2011; Paradis et al. 2014; Reeves et al. 2017b).

UNDERSTANDING HOW LOCAL CONTEXT IMPACTS COLLABORATION

Across the globe, limited progress with enhancements in patient safety, combined with inconsistent results from interprofessional QI initiatives (Austin & Provonost, 2015; Centers for Disease Control and Prevention, 2016; Organisation for Economic Co-operation and Development, 2016) is driving interest in greater examination of how local context influences the success or failure of these activities.

Kaplan and colleagues' (2011) seminal article related to quality, includes an evidence-based conceptual model, known as the Model for Understanding Success in Quality (MUSIQ), that explicates twenty-five contextual factors thought to impact QI intervention success. MUSIQ categorises factors based on their level of operation within the healthcare delivery system and focuses on the following: external environment; organisation; microsystem and team (Kaplan et al. 2011). Examples of the factors at each level include regulatory requirements and competition (external environment), leadership and resource availability (organisation), unit culture and motivation to change (microsystem), and leadership and decision-making process (team). Kaplan et al. (2011) go on to hypothesise that team-based factors (e.g. clinician team leadership behaviour needed to successfully implement improvements at the bedside) directly influence the outcome of collaborative QI projects, whereas other factors (e.g. organisational support), exert an indirect influence on team behaviour.

Kringos et al. (2015) used MUSIQ to frame a systematic review of the literature that explored evidence-based associations between contextual factors and QI intervention success. Further, Kaplan et al. (2013) conducted a cross-sectional survey of participants involved in QI interventions (n = 74) to quantitatively test interrelationships among the twenty-five contextual factors. Findings from this review and other studies discussed suggest that team leadership, team skills, and organisational resource support play important roles in the success of quality-focused interprofessional interventions (Kringos et al. 2015).

In the specific context of interprofessional teamwork, Reeves et al. (2010) identified four domains, and associated domain-specific sub-factors, known to influence the quality of collaborative teamwork: relational, processual, organisational, and contextual (Figure 0.1). Viewed collectively, the sub-factors are all interprofessional issues critical care team members may experience daily in delivering care (Reeves et al. 2016). Sub-factors may be overt, such as the presence or absence of daily interprofessional rounds, or subtle, such as workload issues that prevent nurses from being able to participate in interprofessional rounds within a critical care context (Kendall-Gallagher et al. 2016).

QI interventions can be designed to incorporate important social contextual factors known to impact critical care outcomes. For example, Dixon-Woods et al. (2011) provided a detailed analysis of how an evidenced-based clinical protocol designed to reduce central venous catheter blood stream infections (CVC-BSI) can be developed purposively to address social contextual factors that potentially enhance the opportunity for successful and sustainable improvement. The QI intervention, known as the Michigan Keystone Project that involved 103 ICUs (Pronovost et al. 2006, 2010), facilitated clinician behaviour change through a combination of a structured protocol that included empowering nurses to stop catheter insertion if the clinical protocol was not being followed. It also reframed CVC-BSI as a social problem that could be improved through "human action and behaviour" rather than as "a problem with a simple technical fix" (Dixon-Woods et al. 2011, p. 183).

Bion and colleagues (2012) attempted to replicate the success of the Michigan CVC-BSI initiative in a government-initiated patient safety intervention in over 200 ICUs in England. Results from this study indicated a substantial reduction in reported CVC-BSI in adult ICUs (Bion et al. 2012). However, a more detailed review of study data suggested that "concurrent and preceding improvement efforts" rather than the safety intervention may have accounted for the results (Bion et al. 2012, p. 8). Findings from a related ethnographic study by Dixon-Wood et al. (2013) of seventeen of the participating ICUs in the Bion et al. (2012) study suggested that differences in context play a pivotal role in program outcomes. Identified differences in context included a local peer-driven versus government-driven program, lack of participant engagement due to previous experience with other initiatives and availability of high quality data collection systems (Dixon-Woods et al. 2013).

Collectively, the critical care literature effectively demonstrates that local context (and local cultures) need to be paid close and detailed attention to when studying collaboration or intervening to improve the delivery of inter-professional care.

CREATING PSYCHOLOGICALLY SAFE ENVIRONMENTS

Psychological safety is about interpersonal risk-taking in the workplace (Edmondson, 1999). In a critical care context, Manthous & Hollingshead (2011) describe psychological safety as "a culture in which it is safe for all members to offer their observations and opinions, especially when germane to the quality of delivered care and patient safety" (p. 19). Lack of psychological safety can lead to missed information that can trigger erroneous decision-making and increased risk of patient harm (Manthous & Hollingshead, 2011). Psychological safety can impact quality of care on multiple levels, including provider behaviour related to reporting of adverse events (Appellebaum et al. 2016) and "engagement in quality improvement work" (Nembhard & Edmondson, 2006, p. 941).

The hierarchical status difference among the health professions frequently impedes positive interprofessional interactions and can undermine psychological safety (e.g. Siedlecki & Hixson, 2015). Quality of communication between nurses and physicians continues to present patient safety concerns (Johnson, 2009). It has been argued that notwithstanding the professional hierarchical issues, interprofessional leaders can create an environment of psychological safety (Manthous & Hollingshead, 2011) and facilitate team learning by modelling leader inclusiveness, defined as the "words and deeds by a leader or leaders that indicate an invitation or appreciation for others' contributions" (Nembhard & Edmondson, 2006, p. 947).

Nembhard and Edmondson (2006) explored how leader inclusiveness of team members could "overcome the inhibiting effects of status differences" (p. 941) in twenty-three neonatal ICUs and found that in interprofessional teams, positive associations existed between the following factors: higher professional status and greater psychological safety; leadership inclusiveness and psychological safety; and psychological safety and engagement in quality improvement, respectively. These authors also found that leader inclusiveness moderated the association between professional status and psychological safety (Nembhard & Edmondson, 2006).

Manthous & Hollingshead (2011) for example advocate that improving patient outcomes in critical care settings will require that interprofessional team leaders, inclusive of nurse managers and attending (senior) physicians, practice three behaviours: cultivate psychological safety for all team members; develop the team's transactive memory capability that allows professions to function cohesively and effectively together overtime in an interdependent and interconnected manner; and demonstrate leadership skills that empower team members, particularly during interprofessional rounds.

While this emerging body of research helpfully elucidates the positive effects of leadership on safety and interprofessional collaboration, additional research is needed to better understand how psychological safety moves from concept to practice within an interprofessional team (Edmondson & Lei, 2014).

GIVING PATIENTS AND THEIR FAMILIES VOICE

Effective collaboration engages patients and their families (Robert Wood Johnson Foundation, 2015). From a conceptual perspective, patient-centred care makes intuitive sense; however, from an operational perspective, the concept is challenging to implement, particularly in the critical care environment where "the nature and extent of patient/family involvement can be fraught with tension" (Olding et al. 2016, p. 1184).

The US Society of Critical Care Medicine recently published its new *Guidelines for Family-Centred Care* that "represent the current state of international science in family-centred care and family support for family members of critically ill patients across the lifespan" (Davidson et al. 2017, p. 104). Family-centred care is defined as "an approach to healthcare that is respectful of and responsive to individual families' needs and values" (Davidson et al. 2017, p. 106). The methods used for guideline development included both scoping and systematic reviews. The scoping review allowed for exploration of the qualitative literature in the context of family-centred care within the critical care setting, while the systematic review provided the quantitative foundation and grading of evidence related to practice recommendations (Davidson et al. 2017). These authors found that the quality of evidence for family-centred care ranged from very low to moderate and covered five topics, "communication with family members, family presence, family support, consultations and ICU team members, and operational and environmental issues" (p. 104). Building on this work Gerritsen et al. (2017) argue for a concerted effort to develop a more robust family-centred evidence base in addition to improving the quality of clinicians' communication with family members. The stress associated with having a family member admitted to a critical care unit is common with an estimated "one-quarter to half of family members of critically ill experiencing significant psychological symptoms . . ." (Gerritsen et al. 2017, p. 550). Quality of communication between healthcare providers and the family combined with inclusion of family members in care and decision-making contribute to better family member outcomes (Davidson et al. 2012).

In a recently published scoping review of the literature related to patient and family involvement in adult critical and intensive care settings, Olding and colleagues (2016) found that much of the literature focused on family involvement as passive recipients of care rather than as active partners. The literature fails to explore professional as well as socio-cultural factors that may enhance or impede patient and family involvement (Fox & Reeves, 2015; Gachoud et al. 2012; Olding et al. 2016).

A growing number of studies are also being published in this area. For example, Reeves and colleagues (2015a) interviewed patients' family members as part of an ethnographic study of interprofessional collaboration and family involvement in four ICUs in the USA and Canada. The interviews revealed that family members play diverse, active roles as translators of medical information for family members, advocates, and providers of care with family members noting the importance of having positive interactions with ICU staff. In addition, Curtis et al. (2016) conducted a study that involved 268 family members of 168 ICU patients at the end of life to determine if a communication facilitator decreased family members' distress. Using validated tools to measure anxiety, depression and post-traumatic stress disorder, the authors found that family depression symptoms were reduced at six months with no other significant findings with the exception of reduced ICU and hospital length of stay for patients who died suggesting that use of communication facilitators may foster end-of-life discussions with family members earlier during a patient's hospital stay (Curtis et al. 2016).

THE ROLE FOR INTERPROFESSIONAL EDUCATION

As noted above, high-quality interprofessional interactions are at the heart of effective collaborative practice. Effective interprofessional education can function as the cornerstone for delivering effective collaboration (e.g. Lutfiyya et al. 2016a). Research has continued to demonstrate that interprofessional education can prepare professionals to engage in collaborative problem-solving with shared decision-making (Reeves et al. 2016). Learning collaborative knowledge and skills occurs along a continuum rather than a point in time (Interprofessional Education Collaborative Expert Panel 2011, 2016), whether the learner is a new health professions student or a seasoned clinician.

Kirkpatrick's (1967) seminal framework for evaluating learner outcomes associated with educational initiatives, later adapted for interprofessional education by Barr et al. (1999) provides a useful roadmap for understanding the IPE learning continuum from Level 1 – Reaction; Level 2a – Modification of attitudes/perceptions; Level 2b – Acquisition of knowledge and/or skills; Level 3 – Behavioural change; Level 4a – Change in organisational practice; and Level 4b – Benefits to patients/clients. This approach to classifying the outcomes generated from IPE has now been used to understand the effects of IPE on its participants and on patient care (e.g. Barr et al. 2005; Reeves et al. 2016).

To improve the current "state of the science" for interprofessional education, it has been argued that strides need to be taken to change the current focus on learner outcomes (levels 1, 2a and 2b) to investigating the longer-term effects of collaborative behaviour, organisational practice and patient outcomes – levels 3, 4a and 4b (Lutfiyya et al. 2016b; Reeves et al. 2016). However, gathering evidence at these levels has proven very challenging to achieve (Lutfiyya et al. 2016a). System barriers that impede the move from awareness of IPECP to behaving differently to achieve interprofessional practice include the complexity of implementing collaborative initiatives, difficulty in measuring initiative-related return on investment and variability in the application of interprofessional concepts and processes (Lutfiyya et al. 2016a; Reeves et al. 2016).

Links between interprofessional education and interprofessional collaboration have been demonstrated at the local level and in specific organisational settings but has not yet been established at the national level (Lutfiyya et al. 2016b). Emerging research suggest that healthcare organisations are beginning to report improvements in interprofessional collaboration in relation to delivery of care, patient and provider satisfaction, quality, and organisational financial performance (e.g. Robert Wood Johnson Foundation, 2015; Reeves et al. 2017b).

CONCLUDING COMMENTS

As indicated in this chapter, the literature indicates that issues linked to infrastructure, context, psychological safety and patient/family member involvement play an important role in a critical care context. Underpinning each of these issues is the need for effective collaboration and communication. Drawing on these issues, the subsequent chapters provide a series of tools and activities which help assess, intervene and gather evidence for change.

CHAPTER 2

Assessing and addressing collaborative practice issues

....

INTRODUCTION

Having outlined some key issues in the literature, this chapter provides a series of activities designed to assess the nature of collaboration between healthcare providers and intervene to enhance the quality of interprofessional collaboration within a critical care setting. The chapter presents three iterative activities. The first two activities (interviews with clinical staff and observations of collaboration) have been designed to gain a deeper understanding of interprofessional dynamics and identify related issues that can contribute to patient harm. Based on data gathered from these activities, the third activity aims to improve interprofessional collaboration and communication to help increase quality and safety of patient care. Finally, the chapter outlines some ideas for evaluation of these activities.

PART 1: ASSESSMENT OF INTERPROFESSIONAL COLLABORATION ISSUES

To accurately assess the nature of interprofessional activities two key types of data need to be gathered: interviews and observations. This part of the chapter initially discusses the need for undertaking interviews of critical care staff to gather their perceptions on collaboration. The next part of the chapter discusses the need for gathering observational data to record actual inter-professional collaboration processes.

Interviews

Gathering interview data is vital in any assessment of interprofessional colla-boration as it provides some important insights into the nature of how staff *perceive* what is occurring in a critical care setting in relation to successes and challenges. Interviews can also provide evidence for the different meanings staff attach to collaboration as well as an indication of the values and attitudes they hold about collaboration. Most significantly, gathering interview data is import-ant as perceptual accounts provide an insight into how individuals actually see or experience their world. As such, perceptions provide personal truths.

Interviewer selection

The selection of an interviewer is important as their identity can affect what kind of information healthcare professionals are willing to share (Coar & Sim, 2006). There are two basic types of interviewer to consider:

The insider

Someone being interviewed may develop a better rapport with an interviewer who shares a similar professional background and experience (i.e. an 'insider') and may be more likely to disclose controversial or private views. However, a presumed understanding of issues between two healthcare professionals may prevent new insights.

The outsider

This status as a non-clinician may prompt staff to explain these 'taken-for-granted' team dynamics in greater detail, but this status may also foster sus-picion and reticence.

The advantages and disadvantages of different interviewer backgrounds, as well as available resources, should be considered and discussed when selecting an interviewer. For example, it may be more expensive to engage an outsider, but there may be workload implications for an insider who works on the unit.

Examples of interviewers:

- advanced practice nurse (e.g. clinical nurse specialist or nurse educator),
- social worker,
- other critical care staff member with qualitative interviewing skills,
- graduate student,
- external researcher.

Selecting staff to be interviewed

In order to learn how clinical staff understand interprofessional collaboration, it is important to talk to a range of different professions working in the critical care unit as well as those who hold administrative, leadership, and/or managerial positions.

The sample size for the assessment will depend on the composition of your unit and organisation. As a rule of thumb, collect data until no new themes or information are emerging from the interviews. In general, 20 per cent participation would be reasonable, ideally with each profession represented.

Include a variety of different care professionals who are involved with patient care in your clinical unit, as well as local administrator, leaders and managers. Include participants with a range of experience working in this and other units. Those who are newer to the team will bring different insights than those who have been around for a longer amount of time. Further advice on conducting interviews can be found in Appendix 3.

Should the interview recordings be transcribed?

Often recorded interviews are transcribed verbatim with identifying interviewee information blacked out. Word-for-word transcription allows there to be a clear audit trail, and can be helpful when analysing the data (Halcomb & Davidson, 2006).

Transcription may not be the best option in all situations because it is expensive, time consuming and takes advanced clerical skills to ensure accuracy (Burns & Grove, 2009). Interviewers can transcribe their own interviews, or they can use a combination of taking notes during the interview and audio recording for future reference (Halcomb & Davidson, 2006).

Interview schedule

When developing an interview schedule there are a number of elements to consider:

Introduction

When the participant arrives, introduce yourself and explain why they are being interviewed. Below are possible introductory scripts for an *outsider* and an *insider* interviewer. See Box 2.1.

QUESTIONS

The following questions may be of use to guide an interview with a critical care staff member:

1 What is your role in this unit?
2 Which other healthcare professionals do you interact with, and in what ways?
3 How would you describe interprofessional collaboration in the unit?
4 From your perspective, what are the main responsibilities of: nurses; physicians; respiratory therapists; social workers; occupational therapists; dieticians, etc.?
5 How do you think other healthcare professionals would describe your role in this unit?

BOX 2.1 Possible introductions to use before interviewing

Outsider:

> Hello, my name is [interviewer's name] and I am a [interviewer's position] at [interviewer's institution]. You have been approached to speak with us today because you are a healthcare professional in this unit. We are interested to learn more about how healthcare professionals understand the roles and responsibilities of different healthcare professionals in the team. We are not trying to evaluate your techniques, experience or competencies as a healthcare professional. Rather, we are trying to learn about your perspective on the team, which will hopefully inform future initiatives to improve teamwork and patient safety. In this interview, I will ask you questions about . . .

Insider:

> Hello, my name is [interviewer's name]. As you may know, I am [interviewer's position] in the unit. Right now we're talking to various healthcare professionals to gain insight into how our team understands each other's roles and responsibilities. We wanted to talk to you because of your role as a [interviewee's profession] on our unit. The purpose of this interview is not to evaluate you, and any views you express in this interview will remain confidential. Rather, we are trying to learn about your perspective on the team, which will hopefully inform future initiatives to improve teamwork and patient safety. In this interview, I will ask you questions about . . .

Conclusion

Finish by thanking the participant for taking the time to speak with you, and let them know of any additional steps or contact you may have with them.

Interpreting the results

Review your transcripts or notes/recordings to extrapolate information on whom the staff consider to be collaborating, as well as the various perspectives on the roles of different professions. These findings can be mapped into the matrices tables below (Miles & Huberman, 1994). These tables are a way to analyse qualitative research data by clustering related items into rows and columns (Onwuegbuzie & Dickinson, 2008).

These tables will help identify any trends in how healthcare professionals define and understand interprofessional collaboration in your unit.

Perception of roles matrix.
This matrix compares how healthcare professionals conceptualise their role versus how other professional groups conceptualise it. Below is an example of a partially filled out matrix using data from the study that informed the workbook. Depending on your unit, you may have different healthcare professionals listed in this matrix (see Table 2.1).

Triangulation of perspectives on roles
This matrix compares how healthcare professionals perceive their role, how they think others perceive their role, and how others actually perceive their role in the unit. Below is an example of a partially filled out matrix using data from the study that informed the workbook. Depending on your unit, you may have different healthcare professionals listed in this matrix (see Table 2.2).

Who is in the critical care team?
Table 2.3 provides one way of mapping out how various professionals conceptualise the nature of interprofessional collaboration in the critical care unit. Depending on your unit, you may have different healthcare professionals listed in this matrix.

Applying the PROC framework
Another way to understand the data collected is to apply the four domains of the PROC framework when analysing your transcripts or notes/recordings. As previously noted, the framework has framed interprofessional teamwork by using the following domains:

- Relational factors which affect the relationships shared by professions.
- Processual factors which affect how the work processes are carried out by team members.
- Organisational factors that affect the local environment in which a team is situated.
- Contextual factors (social, political and economic) that affect a team's performance.

The use of this framework allows individuals to consider factors that are a part of their working environment and their effects on the delivery of care. This will allow staff to gain a deeper understanding of their cultural context, and identify areas that can contribute to increased patient risk.

TABLE 2.1 A matrix to compare/contrast differing professional roles

	Nurse perspective	Physician perspective	Physiotherapist perspective	Social worker perspective	Pharmacist perspective
Role of nurses	To care for the patient holistically.	Primary person taking care of the patient.	Point person between all healthcare professionals. Closest to the patient.		Administer medications.
Role of physicians	Leader.	Leader of the team.	Fellows: directs care, manages the unit. Staff: back-up.	Directs team.	Leader.
Role of physiotherapists	Get patient mobilised.	Mobilise patients.			
Role of social workers	Deal with emotional families, family meetings.	Determine POA, locate family, identify John Does.	Talk to families.	Patient advocate. Care for patients and families. Liaison between ICU team and family.	
Role of pharmacists	Communicate medications.	Guardian of medications.			Evaluate drug therapy problems and ensure best practices.

TABLE 2.2 A matrix to recording professional role perceptions

	How they preceive their own role	How they think others perceive their role	How others actually perceive their role
Nurses	To care for the patient holistically.	Primary healthcare professional at the bedside.	Primary person taking care of the patient. Point person between all healthcare professionals. Closest to the patient.
Physicians			
Physiotherapist			
Social worker			
Pharmacist			

TABLE 2.3 An approach to recording professional roles and functions

Profession	Team member role/function
Nurse	
Physician	
Occupational Therapist	
Physiotherapist	
Pharmacist	
Social worker	

Box 2.2 provides two data extracts from the original study to show how the PROC factors can offer different insights into the nature of interprofessional collaboration.

Using the PROC framework as a template to analyse your data can also help by providing categories to help add your data analysis.

By applying the PROC framework, you can better understand some of the underlying issues that are impacting on interprofessional teamwork and patient care in your unit. Using the PROC framework to analyse your data at this stage can also make it easier to select effective interventions (see Chapter 4).

BOX 2.2 Examples of coded data

The following is a data extract coded as a *relational factor*:

> I read the chart only when I can't get in touch with the person to talk to them. But we, by our nature or by busyness or by something, don't write everything in the chart and the nurses don't write everything in the chart. And so, if you ask them what happened in the half hour before the person got intubated, they can tell you in precise detail and they know if they suctioned or not or gave meds or not or turned the patient or what. They'll know all that but it won't be written down because that's not how our charting is designed to be recorded. So talking to the source I find you get better precision because with any oral history . . . Well, even when I tell you a story and you tell your friend and they tell their friend, the story is going to change a little bit. And we certainly have broken telephone at times in medicine, right, but the closer you are to the first story teller the more accurate your information tends to be.

The following is a data extract coded as a *contextual factor*:

> There are political factors involved in deferring to families. As government funding for hospitals has decreased, hospitals are increasingly dependent on the foundation to raise money for their day-to-day functioning which means hospitals are very sensitive to how they are perceived in the press and how they are perceived in the courts. And how they are perceived to any patient family that may be a potential donor whether large or small, and for better or worse that now plays a large role in how we interact with patient families which is the cynical side to patient-family-centred care.

TABLE 2.4 Possible themes and subthemes

Theme	Possible subthemes
Relational	• Hierarchical relations • Unclear team roles
Processual	• Limited time for communication • Ritualised behaviours
Organisational	• Management support for collaboration • Clinical unit differences
Contextual	• Gender issues • Profession-specific cultures

Next steps

The findings from the interviews will be very useful in the intervention activities (Part 2 of this chapter) to address any issues related to collaboration identified. However, these data can be presented to colleagues during a staff meeting to keep them updated on progress with this part of the assessment work.

Observations

Observation is a systematic approach to observing and describing events, activities, people and interactions within a social setting. These data are now used widely in social and health science research to examine the nature of professional and interprofessional interactions and exchanges. Within a critical care context, the purpose of observation is to identify how healthcare professionals interact in practice, both within and between professional groups.

As previously mentioned, interview data provide important perceptual accounts of collaboration. However, such perceptions do not always provide a valid (i.e. enacted) insight of practice. Indeed, there can be a discrepancy between interview and observational data as has been reported in the literature – where professionals' interviews about their perceptions of the clinical unit as having good levels of collaboration were not supported by the observational data (e.g. Reeves & Lewin, 2004; Reeves et al. 2009). This is where the use of observations is needed – to provide an accurate source of evidence into the collaborative practices that actually occur.

Who should gather observational data?

Similar to collecting interview data, the perceived identity of the observer will have implications on the kind of information that healthcare professionals share with you.

Insider

The people being observed may develop a better rapport with an observer who shares a similar professional background and experience (i.e. an 'insider'). However, it is important for 'insiders' to be aware of their own assumptions and make an effort to ask for explanations, even though they may feel that the answer is obvious.

Outsider

An observer from outside the healthcare organisation may garner more detailed information about interprofessional collaboration and roles, since 'taken-for-granted' assumptions about roles and division of labour will need to be explained in greater detail. Additionally, an outsider will take less for granted, and thus ask for more explanation.

It is also important to consider how clinical authority could alter staff behaviours and clinical practices. For example, the unit manager would not be an ideal observer.

What activities should be observed?

- Interprofessional interactions – interactions between professional groups.
- Intraprofessional interactions – interactions within professional groups.
- Formal events – rounds, family conferences.
- Informal events – coffee/tea breaks, impromptu conversations in corridors.

How much should be observed?

Ideally, observation will continue until no new or relevant information is revealed (data saturation), but given the condensed nature of this exercise, observation will be complete once the questions below are satisfactorily answered (approximately 20 hours over a two-week period during mornings, afternoons and evenings). Ensure the observations are on different days and times (including day and night shifts) so you can capture the variety of issues encountered by many different staff members.

Areas to focus observation on

The following three areas are important to focus on when undertaking observational work:

1 Who interacts with whom?
   - When and how often?
   - Who interacts the most/the least?
   - What kinds of interactions take place (e.g. rapid, lengthy, clinical/social content)?

2 Where do interprofessional interactions take place?

- – Between whom?
- – What kinds of interactions take place?

3 Where do intraprofessional interactions take place?

- – Between whom?
- – What kinds of interactions take place?

Field notes

Writing up

Writing up detailed notes is an integral part of observation, and should ideally occur soon after a period of observation to maximise the accuracy of recall. When writing up field notes, the researcher will want to keep the following two elements separate (description and impression) – see Table 2.5.

When writing up field notes, refer to individuals by their role and profession rather than their name. When necessary to distinguish a particular individual, use pseudonyms to protect anonymity. The aim of observation should be to identify patterns in interaction and teamwork rather than single out individual behaviour.

Further guidance about collecting observations, including an example of an observational field note can be found in Appendix 4.

Interpreting the results

Analysing field notes is an iterative process that begins while you are still in the observation phase (Reeves et al. 2013). As you continually review your field notes, you will begin to notice emerging themes, such as which groups interact the most. These emerging themes can help shape when and where you do more observations.

TABLE 2.5 Organising the analysis of data

What it is	Example
Description of events: A non-evaluative description of what happened	"Person x gave a report on the patient's status, which was interrupted three times by person y"
Impressions: The observer's impressions of events, including their feelings and sense of emerging patterns	"I felt like the contributions of person x were not valued in the rounds"

As you are reviewing the field notes, also make note of any observations or insights that begin to emerge (Burns & Grove, 2009; Onwuegbuzie & Dickinson, 2008). This may help clarify your ideas, help connect concepts, and will help you remember any insights that you had. The information gathered at this stage will be presented to critical care staff during the subsequent Interprofessional Collaboration Workshop.

Using the PROC framework as a template to analyse your data will provide a number of categories to add your data into (i.e. relational factors, processual factors, organisational factors and contextual factors) which can help with the generation of themes and subthemes related to the data (see Table 2.4).

Like the analysis of interview data, use of the PROC framework in the analysis of the observations may also make it easier to select effective interventions (see Chapter 4).

Next steps

The observations will be very useful in the intervention activities (Part 2 of this chapter) to address any issues related to collaboration identified. However, similar to the use of the interview data, these data can be presented to colleagues during a staff meeting to keep them updated on progress of the assessment work.

PART 2: INTERVENTIONS TO IMPROVE INTERPROFESSIONAL COLLABORATION

Once you have gathered and analysed your interview and observational data it is time to share it with your critical care colleagues. The first activity to consider is an initial workshop that can provide critical care staff with an overview of the key findings from the observations and interviews, as well as exploring their own perceptions of interprofessional collaboration. This part of the chapter goes on to also offer some additional ideas for follow-up activities to help both disseminate and take action on the findings from the interviews and observations.

Workshop

This initial workshop can be integrated into a pre-existing meeting on a critical care unit as a compressed 45–60-minute activity, or run separately over a longer period, for example 2–3 hours. It is very likely that not all staff will be able to attend a single workshop. As a result, this initial session will likely need to be offered on a number of occasions to ensure as many critical care professionals as possible can participate. Also, consider whether there are any learning activities that can be 'flipped' – where participants can be sent materials to review/read ahead of the workshop – this can help ensure that there is more time for active learning during the workshop.

Below are some ideas about possible learning outcomes, workshop content and facilitation.

Learning outcomes and contents

Effective delivery of any educational activity requires clear and achievable learning outcomes. Given the focus of the data collection activities described above, the following learning outcomes will be useful to employ – see Box 2.3.

In terms of the contents of this initial workshop, the following activities, offered in three sections, with a fourth optional section, are suggested:

1 Exploring the nature of interprofessional work

   As an icebreaking activity, the workshop could begin with asking participants to list all of the different healthcare professionals they work with and then encouraging them to discuss and record the dynamics that occur between these professions.

2 Share key findings from the interviews and observations

   An interactive presentation can be undertaken to highlight key findings from the observations and interviews. This can be done by selecting some of the analysed data from matrices, or anonymous quotes/vignettes to share with participants. Throughout the presentation, the facilitator should spark reaction and discussion around the selected data by asking the participants how these findings resonate with their own individual experiences of interprofessional collaboration.

3 Create an interactions chart

   Following the interactive presentation and discussion, the facilitator should encourage participants to revisit the list of professionals and dynamics created in the first part of the workshop. Participants can arrange the different professions to depict the flows of collaboration and communication that occur within their unit.

4 Selecting interventions to improve collaboration – Optional

   Depending on the participants and facilitator, this workshop may be an appropriate time to start a discussion around what kind of intervention(s) would be most appropriate to address this issues that have been uncovered by the collection of the interviews and observations.

   However, before selecting any intervention(s) it would be appropriate to first complete the activities in Chapter 4 to further explore staff perceptions of which PROC framework issues are the priority in their unit. Chapter 4 also contains a list of different types of interventions that can be used to address these concerns.

**BOX 2.3 Possible learning outcomes
(improving collaboration workshop)**

By the end of this workshop, participants will be able to:

1 List healthcare professionals in their critical care unit and describe how they work together.
2 Explain key elements from the findings of the observations and interviews completed on their unit.
3 Apply learning to creating an "interaction chart" (see below).
4 Critique interprofessional collaboration and communication in their unit.

Workshop facilitation

Successful workshop facilitation requires skill, experience and preparation. Barr et al. (2005) have outlined a range of helpful attributes required for effective interprofessional workshop facilitation, including:

- experience of interprofessional critical care work;
- in-depth understanding of interactive learning;
- knowledge of group dynamics;
- confidence in working with interprofessional groups;
- flexibility (to creatively use professional differences within groups).

It is therefore important that a suitably qualified individual is located. For example, an experienced and respected healthcare professional from the critical care unit or a nearby unit, or a representative from the hospital's patient safety or quality improvement unit.

Workshop facilitators need to focus on creating a supportive and safe learning environment, and enabling all participants to have the opportunity to participate equally. Another core skill of an interprofessional facilitator then becomes the ability to make explicit for participants, learning moments which can surface the traditional power hierarchies amongst the professions.

More details on facilitating this workshop can be found in Appendix 5. In addition, more general facilitation guidance is offered in Appendix 9.

Follow-up activities

Following the delivery of the initial workshop, there are a number of other activities to consider to ensure the data gathered from the interviews and observations continue to be used and also to ensure that any decisions taken about further action to improve interprofessional collaboration are being implemented. Below are a number of possible options:

- If there is continued interest, follow-up workshops should be offered to check in with progress on agreed actions to improve interprofessional collaboration.
- Poster(s) summarising the findings from the workshop(s) can be displayed in high-traffic areas so all staff members can see the results (e.g. nursing station, medication room, staff change rooms, or the staff break room).
- The findings from workshop(s) should be presented at staff meetings to help ensure that the focus on assessing and improving interprofessional collaboration continues to be a key area of interest for critical care staff.
- Presentation(s) should be offered to other critical care units in the hospital, as well as the hospital's patient safety and/or quality improvement unit to share workshop findings and achievements with these staff.
- Presentation(s) of workshop findings should be offered to senior management to provide opportunities to engage with key decision makers.

PART 3: EVALUATION

Following the delivering of any intervention activities (e.g. initial workshop(s), follow-up activities) efforts should be made to gather evaluation evidence. Such evidence is an important part of implementing interventions and it provides vital information on the effectiveness (or not) of any intervention.

There are many ways one can gather data to help measure the outcomes and impact of intervention activities. For example, following the initial workshop one can evaluate:

- Shifts in professionals' attitudes towards one another and/or value attached to interprofessional collaboration (surveys).
- Changes in perceptions about interprofessional collaboration (interviews, focus groups).
- Changes in collaborative behaviour between staff (observations).

See Chapter 5 for more information on potential evaluation approaches, methods and data collection tools which can be employed for evaluation work.

CONCLUDING COMMENTS

This chapter has outlined a series of activities designed to assess the collaborative work undertaken by critical care staff. It also offered a series of intervention activities designed to address any identified issues with collaboration. Finally, the chapter provided a range of ideas for evaluating any of the intervention activities.

CHAPTER 3

Collaboration with patients and family members

·····································

INTRODUCTION

This chapter presents a series of activities to allow critical care staff to reflect upon their own understanding about patient/family involvement, and to make them aware of the range of possible definitions of involvement offered by patients/family members. Based upon this reflection activity, the chapter also describes an intervention focused on facilitating a direct approach for patients/family members to convey to professionals their desired level of involvement. In doing so, the chapter aims to provide a more nuanced view of the range of what involvement means to family members themselves. Finally, the chapter offers a range of suggestions to evaluate these activities.

WHAT WE KNOW ABOUT FAMILY INVOLVEMENT

Research on best practices for family member involvement has shown that such involvement improves care quality in critical care settings and helps to reduce medical errors leading to adverse events. While many critical care units promote the principle of "patient-centred care" and family member involvement, there can be a significant gap between knowledge about these processes and their translation into practice. Among the reasons for this challenge is the lack of research on the experiences of family members within the day-to-day critical care context. Additionally, few studies have explored the different ways in which "patient and family involvement" is defined by clinicians themselves, in diverse groups such as nurses, physicians, and other health professionals.

As outlined in the introduction, the research upon which this chapter is based has found that the concept of patient-centred care is not uncontroversial among healthcare providers. While the different hospitals in the study had varying degrees of institutional commitment to promoting patient-centred care (for example, in the form of strategic plans and hospital mandates), at the clinical level, the meaning and form of its practice were largely up for individual interpretation. Family involvement can be a sensitive topic, and when probed for its meaning, healthcare providers offered a range of responses. This was not entirely surprising, given how differently family involvement impacts different healthcare professionals. Nurses, for instance, are most directly impacted by the presence and involvement of family members in the delivery of care, whereas physicians often described family involvement in terms of decision-making, and the related potential legal implications. This is also reflected in the literature.

In research from Europe and North America, family presence is positively associated to patient care – a fact also acknowledged by frontline staff (e.g. Chiang, 2011; Olsen et al. 2009; Söderström et al. 2009), but yet remains largely informal, thus often being left to nurse discretion (Kean & Mitchell, 2013; McConnell & Moroney, 2015). Clearly, challenges exist related to the formalisation of guidelines, ranging from healthcare provider attitudes toward patient-centred care (Agård & Maindal, 2009; Kean & Mitchell, 2013) to practical and logistical considerations (Agård & Lomborg, 2011; Fulbrook et al. 2005). A central issue, it seems, is not the inability of hospitals to formulate and institute family involvement policies and guidelines, but rather the cultural resistance to the formalisation of such rules in the first place. The lack of such guidelines – or more commonly, the lack of their enforcement – has left the interpretation and practice of family involvement largely up to frontline staff. Research has shown that this is problematic for both patients and their families (e.g. Black et al. 2011; Blom et al. 2013; Broyles et al. 2012; Mitchell & Chaboyer, 2010; Sullivan et al. 2012).

The challenge, it seems, lies not in formulating or instituting such policies, but rather in grappling with the cultural acceptance of this approach. Interventions to promote "patient-centred care" and family involvement must address the local meanings and implications for the various healthcare providers – for we know from our research that the meanings and implications of patient-centred care and family involvement vary across different healthcare professionals. For instance, while at the institutional level, an open visitation policy may be a direct reflection of established values of incorporating family members as part of the care team, the realisation of this practice may provoke concerns from frontline staff related to surveillance and delivery of care. Similarly, loosely defined pledges to encourage family involvement raise the question of appropriate roles and can be perceived as threatening the current level of practical discretion allowed to healthcare providers.

PART 1: ASSESSING THE NATURE OF PATIENT/FAMILY MEMBER INVOLVEMENT

Similar to the assessment of interprofessional collaboration in Chapter 2, to help accurately assess the nature of patient/family member involvement in a critical care unit, it is recommended that observations are initially undertaken. These data can be used with a second activity focused on defining family member involvement designed to help critical care staff gain a deeper insight into family involvement in the delivery of care.

Observations

As previously noted, observational data can be very useful for generating rich descriptions of events, activities and interactions. Indeed, this form of data can offer direct evidence into how family members are actually involved (or not) in the care of their relatives.

Approach

Similar to the guidance offered in the previous chapter, the perceived identity of the observer will have implications on the kind of information that family members share with you. Therefore, thought is needed about whether to employ an 'insider' or an 'outsider' to gather these data.

What activities should be observed?

- Interactions – between patients/family members and staff;
- formal events – patient/family conferences;
- informal events – impromptu patient/family member-staff conversations.

How much should be observed?

As previously noted, observations, ideally, should continue until data saturation is achieved, but given the condensed nature of this activity, observation will be complete once the questions below are satisfactorily answered (approximately 20 hours over a two-week period during mornings, afternoons and evenings). Ensure the observations are on different days and times (including day and night shifts) so you can capture the variety of issues linked to family member involvement.

Areas to focus observation on

The following three areas are important to concentrate on when undertaking family member involvement observations:

1 Who (patient/family member) interacts with whom (staff member)?

   - When and how often?

   – Who interacts the most/the least?
   – What kind of interactions take place (e.g. rapid, lengthy, nature of content)?

2 Where do patient/family member interactions take place?

   – Between whom?
   – What kind of interactions take place?

3 Why do these interactions take place?

Field notes

Like the guidance offered in the previous chapter the following issues need to be paid attention to:

- Ideally occur soon after a period of observation to maximise the accuracy of recall.
- When writing up field notes, the researcher will want descriptions and impressions separate (see Table 2.5).
- When writing up field notes, refer to individuals by their role (e.g. patient's daughter) rather than their name.
- When necessary to distinguish a particular individual, use pseudonyms to protect anonymity.
- Further guidance about collecting observations, including an example of an observational field note can be found in Appendix 4.

Interpreting the results

Issues to consider when interpreting (analysing) the data:

- Given the iterative nature of observational work data collection and analysis proceed simultaneously
- Continually review field notes to look for emerging themes/issues linked to family involvement
- Make notes of emergent trends/patterns in the observations as these can be used in the family member involvement workshop (below) or presented to colleagues during a staff meeting to keep them updated on progress of this work.

PART 2: UNDERSTANDING FAMILY MEMBER PERSPECTIVES ABOUT INVOLVEMENT

This activity involves a process to help critical care staff gain a deeper understanding of the variation in how families choose to be involved in the delivery of care and become more aware of their own understanding of family involvement in the delivery of care.

To help 'set the scene' for this activity, below are some real-life examples (taken from the ICU study interviews) of how family members have expressed their desired level of involvement:

I am an advocate for my dad. I like to know what his stats are, and get detailed information about how he is doing. I have a lot of questions, and also research his medical condition online when I have time.

I am here for support. My husband feels scared without me. I try to be here as much as I can, but do not want to hear about all the medical details. I leave that to the doctors.

I have been my sister's primary caregiver for the past 10 years. I am used to taking care of her medical needs, and would like to be involved in any way I can. I have a lot of information about her condition and medications she takes at home. I am very involved in her care.

I am here to spend time with my mom. I come when I can, but I prefer to check in by phone.

In addition, observational field note extracts (again from the ICU study) are presented below to show how family involvement was regarded in daily clinical work:

At bed 4, the senior RN is explaining the care plan and nutrition to the family member, using very graphic description of feeding tube. He explains the doctors are using it "to give him more nutrition." The family member responds, "as long as he doesn't feel a thing – do what needs to be done. I just want to see him walk out of here."

A physician noted, "you have the patient on this drug, so the family Googles it. And they'll come back with all these questions. And then, you have to really break it down into non-medical terms so they understand what you're doing."

The nurse is walking by and notices that the patient's wife is trying to suction him. She approaches and the wife says, "I'm just trying to ..." and gestures to her neck. The nurse says that she can do it.

A physician comments, "The report I got on days is that she is a little less winded." Another physician makes notes in the chart. The nurse says, "The family is concerned that it's cancer. Something else is brewing. They keep asking about cancer and her lungs."

"I have a patient right now, they're from two and a half hours away, and they call once a day. They don't call ten times a day, which is nice. That really helps because it's a reminder because you're dealing with the patient and the family is not in the room, so you almost lose sight of that sometimes."

Purpose

Given the differences of family member involvement presented in the real-life examples above, it is important to adopt a systematic process for identifying discrepancies between how various family members define the involvement in the care of their loved ones. The activity has been designed to be simple and easy to implement, but will allow family members to convey to staff what their desired level of involvement in the delivery of care is.

Importantly, this activity generates key insights from families that critical care staff can use to reflect, collectively and critically, upon their own understanding about family involvement and acknowledge the range of possible definitions of involvement offered by patients' families.

Implementing family involvement activity

This activity aims to allow family members to communicate (in writing) their desired level of involvement in daily care. The family spokesperson (or other primary caregiver) is provided with a *Family Involvement Record*, which allows them to express in their own words how they define their involvement in the care of their loved one (see Box 3.1).

Instructions for implementation

Below are a number of suggestions to help implement this activity:

- Provide a suitable range of materials, including writing instruments, paper and boards for the family member to write on.
- Ensure you are approaching the family member at an appropriate time.
- Explain that the *Family Involvement Record* is an opportunity for them to express how they define their involvement in the care of their loved one. They can explain how they define their role and how involved they want (or do not want) to be in the delivery of care).
- If they agree, allow the family member time alone to write down their thoughts, views and perspectives on their own. But it is a good idea to agree a time to return.

BOX 3.1 An example of a Family Involvement Record

Family Involvement Record

Instructions for family members

The purpose of this record is to allow family members and caregivers to communicate their desired level of involvement in daily care. This will help healthcare providers better understand your needs. Please use this card to express in your own words how you would like to be involved in the care of your loved one. Add all comments in the space below:

- Once patients leave the unit, collect all *Family Involvement Records* and keep them together. These records will be used in Part 3 – Interventions to improve family involvement (below).

Some ideas for success

Below are a few ideas to help ensure the successful completion of this activity:

1 Using the *Family Involvement Record*
   You may require consent from the patient and/or family member to use this record beyond the patient's stay. Please review your institution's ethical and governance policies before implementing the *Family Involvement Record*.
2 Involve existing personnel and representatives
   Depending on your unit and organisation, you may have access to personnel whose roles are heavily rooted in the family realm, such as patient/family representatives or social workers. You could consult these individuals, as appropriate/applicable for your unit.
3 Displaying the Record
   With the family's permission, you may want to display the *Family Involvement Record*. Possible display locations include: unit walls, bedside whiteboards, and bedside nurse's station. Before displaying the *Family Involvement Record*, consult your unit's policies regarding posting anything

on the walls. Care should of course also be taken to maintain privacy. While the record should be visible to healthcare professionals, it should not be blatantly visible to the visitors of other patients.

PART 3: INTERVENTIONS TO IMPROVE FAMILY INVOLVEMENT

To share key findings from the observations, discuss the findings from the *Family Involvement Record* as well as explore professional views of family involvement, it is proposed that a workshop is offered to critical care staff. Building on the activities from this workshop, the chapter goes on to also offer some additional ideas for a series of follow-up activities to help both disseminate and take action on any agreed actions.

Staff workshop

This workshop allows healthcare professionals to learn more about patient/ family involvement in their critical care unit. This workshop can be integrated into a pre-existing meeting on a critical care unit as a compressed 60-minute activity, or run separately over a longer period, for example 2–3 hours. If not all staff are able to attend the workshop due to time pressures, it can be offered on other occasions to ensure as many staff as possible can participate. Also, consider whether there are any learning activities that can be 'flipped' (sent to participants ahead of the workshop to review/read) as this can help ensure more time is dedicated to active learning.

Learning outcomes and contents

Box 3.2 presents a series of possible learning outcomes for the family involvement workshop.

BOX 3.2 Possible learning outcomes for family involvement workshop

By the end of this workshop, participants will be able to:

- Describe different ways in which family members describe their involvement in their loved one's care.
- Compare differences and similarities in how family members and healthcare professionals understand family involvement.
- Analyse how expectations of family member involvement impact their work.
- Critique practices pertaining to family member involvement in their critical care unit.

Activity 1: Sharing the findings from the observations

This first activity focuses on presenting key findings into the actual real-world practice of how family members are involved (or not) in the care of their loved ones. An interactive presentation can be undertaken to highlight key findings from the observations by using some of the ideas presented above (see Part 2 of Chapter 2).

Activity 2: Reviewing completed *Family Involvement Records*

The purpose of this activity is for participants to reflect on how family members describe their involvement in the delivery of care using the *Family Involvement Records* that were previously collected (see Part 1).

At the workshop, small groups can review the *Family Involvement Records* and discuss what kinds of involvement family members and caregivers have expressed. The small groups can write the key findings onto sticky notes. Then the whole group comes together to arrange all of the findings into themes on the wall. The participants can be asked to reflect on how these findings resonate with their professional practice, and what impact these kinds of involvement have on their work.

More details on facilitating this workshop can be found in Appendix 6. In addition, more general facilitation guidance is offered in Appendix 9.

Follow-up activities

Following the delivery of this workshop, there are a number of other activities to consider ensuring data gathered from the observations and results from the workshop can be used and also to ensure that any decisions taken about further action to improve family member involvement are being implemented. Similar to the follow-up activities presented in Chapter 2, possible options include:

- the delivery of follow-up workshop(s);
- poster(s) summarising the findings from workshop(s);
- presentation of workshop(s) findings to critical care colleagues, other interested hospital staff and senior management.

PART 4: EVALUATION

Evaluation is an important part of implementing interventions to ensure effectiveness. There are many ways you can measure the outcomes of this tool, such as:

- Run the workshop again, and assess for changes in healthcare professionals' thoughts and attitudes between both sessions.

- Observation of unit staff behaviour and uptake of the *Family Involvement Record.*
- Interviews or focus groups.
- Surveys (online or paper-based).
- Areas of assessment in your evaluation may include:

  - Uptake of the Patient/*Family Involvement Record* into practice.
  - Changes in healthcare professionals' perception of family member involvement in the delivery of care.
  - Increased family member involvement integrated into clinical practice.

- Barriers and facilitators for increasing family member involvement in your critical care unit.

See Chapter 5 for more information on potential approaches, methods and tools for the evaluation phase.

CONCLUDING COMMENTS

This chapter described a range of activities designed to encourage critical care staff to reflect upon their own understanding about patient/family involvement, and to make them aware of different definitions of involvement. Based on a careful consideration of the notion of involvement the chapter outlined intervention approaches to help ensure critical care staff actively engaged with patients/family members in the care they delivered. Finally, the chapter outlined a number of suggestions about how to evaluate these activities.

CHAPTER 4

Collaboratively identifying and addressing critical care delivery issues

....

INTRODUCTION

This chapter describes an activity designed to help critical care staff collaboratively identify issues that affect interprofessional collaboration and
patient/family member involvement. Based on the findings of this activity, a
series of interprofessional interventions are offered which aim to improve the
identified issues. The chapter draws on the PROC framework to help address
different processual, relational and organisation factors involved. Collectively,
it is anticipated that engagement in both these activities will allow critical
care staff to gain a deeper understanding of their local culture as well as
identify approaches that can enhance the delivery of effective care.

PART 1: IDENTIFYING CRITICAL CARE ISSUES

This part of the chapter provides details on an activity which aims to engage
with different critical care staff to collaboratively identify the factors that
affect the care they are providing to their patients.

Collaborative critical care workshop

This workshop aims to give critical care staff an opportunity to collaboratively
discuss issues impacting their interprofessional work and its effect on care
delivery in their unit. The overall goal of this workshop is to unveil the root
causes of any identified issues so an effectively tailored, mutually agreed
intervention can be developed. It is anticipated that this activity can be integrated into a pre-existing meeting in the unit (e.g. in-service continuing

education session) as a compressed 45–60 minute activity, or run separately over longer periods as a single or multiple offering – all depending on the availability of staff.

Learning outcomes and contents

The workshop(s) consist of a focused exercise in which critical staff from different professional groups, experience and seniority, collaborate to identify key patient care delivery issues and agree approaches (interventions) which can be implemented to address these issues. Box 3.3 contains a range of possible learning outcomes.

BOX 3.3 Possible learning outcomes – collaborative care workshop

By the end of this workshop, participants will be able to:

- Identify concerns that impact teamwork and/or patient care in the critical care unit.
- Discuss facilitating and restraining forces that contribute to the identified issue.
- Analyse the different levels that are involved in the issue, such as individual healthcare professions, team processes, and the organisation of care.
- Critically reflect on the issue's impact on their clinical practice and patient family members.

Collaborative brainstorming

This activity aims to help healthcare professionals explore interprofessional and patient family issues in their unit using a mind map.[1] For this activity, the map can be organised with a central problem identified by the participants in the middle, and the four components of the PROC framework branching out (see Figure 4.1). Participants can suggest factors influencing the central problem that stem from each of the PROC factors. Using the PROC framework to organise the group's thoughts may make it easier to pick an effective intervention.

The identified problem would be written in the centre box with new ideas branching out from the PROC factors in different colours.

More details on facilitating this workshop can be found in Appendices 7 and 8. In addition, more general facilitation guidance is offered in Appendix 9.

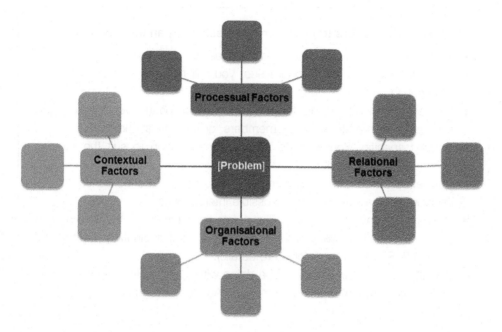

FIGURE 4.1 Collaborative brainstorming using a mind map organised by the PROC framework

PART 2: ADDRESSING CRITICAL CARE ISSUES

Having identified the issues connected with collaboration and patient/family member involvement, the next stage is to consider intervention(s). The focus of this phase is to build on the strengths in your unit to address areas needing improvement. There are a number of factors to consider when selecting and/or designing an intervention – see Box 4.1.

To complement the activity described above, the possible interventions are organised around three of the four domains in the PROC framework (relational, processual and organisational).[2] As well as describing each intervention, we offer some guidance into the frequency, duration and cost of each to help with making informed choices about implementation.

Relational interventions

These interventions involve the use of interprofessional learning activities and should be considered if the workshop discussion uncovers issues such as a need for increased clarity of team roles or discrepancies in critical care staff members' perceptions of patient family involvement. Below is a range of interprofessional activities, which can help resolve relational issues.

BOX 4.1 Factors to consider when selecting an intervention

- Make sure the type of intervention matches the root issue. For example, if you have identified a relational issue, you will need to select a relational intervention.
- You want to ensure you are focusing on the appropriate intervention target, such as team members, family members, or the critical care unit.
- Context specific. You want to tailor the intervention to suit the specific context of your unit setting.
- Cost-effectiveness. It is important to assess cost and effectiveness of the intervention in relation to other possible interventions.
- Evaluation. Consider how you will evaluate the intervention before selecting it. What outcomes will you be measuring? What evaluation method will you use? (See Chapter 5 for more details).
- Results. Consider what you will be doing with your results, and whom you will be disseminating/sharing them with. (Again, see Chapter 5).

Simulation

Simulated learning ranges from low-tech (e.g. role play exercises) to high-tech (e.g. computerised manikins, simulated clinical environments) activities. They can allow professionals to practice near real-life teamwork/family member involvement issues. Simulation can be facilitated by an external facilitator (if resources allow) or delivered by an internal healthcare professional with teaching experience. Ensure time is available for shared reflection (debriefing) at the end of each workshop to review the content of the learning and develop action plans that will be taken back to the critical care unit.

For all types of simulation, develop the scenarios so they are well connected to the findings in the local unit and follow best practices in relation to running the simulation around engagement with learners during the scenarios (e.g. Rosen et al. 2008; Sharma et al. 2011).

FREQUENCY

Depending on the extent of the issues identified in a critical care unit, simulated activities can be offered on a weekly or monthly basis. Providing regular opportunities for simulated activities is recommended to develop and then sustain an active engagement with this form of learning.

DURATION

In general, run a single interprofessional simulation activity for an hour: 20 minutes for the scenario and 40 minutes for the debriefing activity.

COST

Low-tech simulation is an inexpensive option, as it can be developed by healthcare professionals and delivered in seminar rooms near the critical care unit. In contrast, while high-tech simulations are more expensive as simulation labs need to be rented, they may be more appropriate depending on the outcome you are hoping to achieve.

USEFUL RESOURCES

- www.jems.com/article/training/simulation-best-practices
- Leclair et al. (2017) A longitudinal interprofessional simulation curriculum for critical care teams: Exploring successes and challenges.
- www.saferhealthcare.com/crew-resource-management/crew-resource-management-healthcare/

Team reflexivity

A critical care team that spends time together reflecting upon their collaborative work can develop a "reflexive" (e.g. integrated, well-coordinated) way of working together. The development of a reflexive team approach can help ensure that members are able to adapt and respond effectively to any changes they encounter (West, 1996). This is an important quality to have for health and social care teams working together, as change is an on-going factor that needs to be managed by students and staff.

A key aspect to achieving a reflexive approach is the creation of an environment where members value the contributions of all team members, feel safe to openly share their ideas, and trust one another to acknowledge their shortfalls and mistakes.

FREQUENCY

Engaging in a reflexive discussion about interprofessional collaboration and patient/family involvement could be easily included into an existing weekly or monthly staff meeting. A colleague could facilitate the discussion drawing upon identified issues encountered by critical care staff related to collaborative practices involving professionals, patients/families.

DURATION

Around 15–20 minutes of meeting time could be used for a reflexive discussion of collaboration and patient/family involvement issues.

COST

There should be no additional expense needed to implement reflexive discussions if an 'in-house' colleague facilitates the meeting. Expense may however occur if an external facilitator is engaged to deliver this activity.

USEFUL RESOURCES

- Gabelica et al. (2014) The effect of team feedback and guided reflexivity on team performance change.
- www.ideasforleaders.com/ideas/how-team-reflexivity-fosters-innovation
- Konradt et al. (2016) Reflexivity in teams: A review and new perspectives.

Team training

This can consist of interactive workshops where healthcare professionals come together to discuss and problem-solve the issues identified by the mind mapping activity. Such interventions should involve a combination of exploration, examination and reflection aimed at addressing the relational difficulties from the assessment of ICU collaboration and/or family member involvement:

- Develop real-life clinical case(s) linked to the findings from the diagnostics tool.
- Aim to facilitate exploratory discussion of the case(s) from different professional perspectives of all participating healthcare professionals.
- Encourage healthcare professionals to reach a consensus in resolving the case under discussion.
- Ensure time is available for shared reflection at the end of each workshop to review the content of the learning and develop action plans that can be taken back to the ICU.
- Where appropriate, involve patient family members to provide their perspective on the delivery of care.

FREQUENCY

Depending on the extent of the issues identified in the ICU, these workshops may be offered as a single event (with at least a three and six-months follow-up), or offered as a series of weekly or monthly events.

DURATION

To help encourage good attendance, a one-hour time slot is recommended. Look for seminar rooms close to the ICU. If possible offer snacks and refreshments.

COST

To keep costs down, these workshops should be developed and implemented by an internal healthcare professional with experience of small group facilitation.

USEFUL RESOURCES

- http://ipe.utoronto.ca/curriculum/facilitators/tools-resources
- Salas et al. (2008) Does team training improve team performance? A meta-analysis.
- http://healthsciences.curtin.edu.au/faculty/leadership_programme.cfm

Team retreats

If the relational issues identified by the activity required a more in-depth response, a critical care team retreat may be considered. A team retreat would provide staff time to carefully review the collaborative and patient/family member involvement issues that have been identified (away from the on-going distractions of clinical practice).

DURATION

Retreats are usually held for a half-day or full-day. They can be extended to two days (if desired and feasible) depending on the complexity of the issues identified, as well as available resources.

FREQUENCY

Short follow-up meetings should be held at three and six months to discuss progress made since the original retreat.

COST

Costs would need to be set aside for room hire, retreat facilitation, travel and catering. These costs would be extended to include accommodation costs if it was decided to hold a retreat over two days.

USEFUL RESOURCES

- Hills (2003) Organizing a practice retreat.
- http://leadership.uoregon.edu/resources/exercises_tips/events/organize_a_
  retreat
- Clevenger (2007) Improve staff satisfaction with team building retreats.

Team mind mapping

This approach allows the graphic reconstruction of shared team knowledge. Arguably, the increasingly complex task environment in education and work settings combined with high-density information requires new learning and knowledge retention strategies.[1] Mind mapping can therefore by a way of helping organise information via hierarchies or branches. At the centre is an image (concept map, conceptual diagram) displaying the key topic to be explored. Branches labelled with key words indicating major topics associated with the central topic radiate from the central image. This activity may be used by ICU staff to introduce new concepts or explore issues related to their relational work linked to collaboration and family member involvement.[2]

FREQUENCY

Collaborative mind mapping exercises could be easily included into an existing weekly or monthly staff meeting. A colleague could facilitate the exercise during the meeting.

DURATION

Around 15–25 minutes of meeting time could be used for a team-base mind mapping exercise.

COST

There should be no additional expense needed to implement mind mapping if a clinical colleague facilitates the exercise. Expense may however occur if an external facilitator is engaged.

USEFUL RESOURCES

- http://blog.sandglaz.com/use-mind-mapping-unlock-team-creativity/
- Windsor (2013) Using concept mapping in community-based participatory research: a mixed methods approach.
- www.mindjet.com/mind-mapping-project-management/

Interprofessional rounds

Interprofessional rounds are for critical care staff to meet together (often at the bedside) to collaboratively review, plan and agree the care delivered to patients. Growing evidence indicates that the use of interprofessional rounds can enhance collaboration among healthcare providers and improve outcomes (Reeves et al. 2017a). Schwartz Rounds have increasingly been used as a structured forum where clinical and non-clinical, come together (away from the bedside) regularly to discuss the emotional and social aspects of working in healthcare. Their purpose is to understand the challenges and rewards that are intrinsic to providing care, not to solve problems or to focus on the clinical aspects of patient care. They also help to reduce hierarchies between staff and to focus attention on relational aspects of care.

FREQUENCY

Daily interprofessional rounds can be very effective for providing timely collaborative care. If not feasible, weekly interprofessional rounds should be considered. These rounds could be added to an existing profession-specific round if needed.

DURATION

Around 30–60 minutes depending on the number of patients and the severity of their conditions.

COST

No external costs needed to introduce these rounds, though commitment needed to amend staff schedules. A Schwartz Round will need a seminar room and facilitator.

RESOURCES

- Burdick and colleagues (2017) Bedside interprofessional rounding: The view from the patient's side of the bed.
- www.oatext.com/Sharing-the-burden-Schwartz-rounds-as-a-compassion ate-collaborative-practice-and-education-model-in-longterm-care.php
- www.kingsfund.org.uk/projects/schwartz-center-rounds

Family assessment forms

This activity allows family members to describe their connection to the patient and gives the critical care team the opportunity to learn and understand about the patient as an individual within their family. It provides family members with a place to write background information on the patient and their preferences while in a critical care unit. Research has found a family assessment form can shed light on the 'taken-for-granted' assumptions clinical staff may make about families. For example, Blanchard and Alavi (2008) noted that nurses expressed surprise at how kinship was described in their assessment forms by some family members. This form can also act as a reminder for staff to be more inclusive of families.

FREQUENCY

Family assessment forms can be gathered before/after relatives' visits to a critical care unit. The data gathered from these forms can then be included in an existing weekly or monthly staff meeting, where participants review the forms and agree to implement any issues linked to improving family member involvement.

DURATION

Around 10 minutes for a relative to complete the family assessment form, and around 10–30 minutes of staff meeting time (depending on issues identified in form) for reviewing forms and agreeing follow-up actions.

COST

There should be no additional expense needed to implement mind mapping if a clinical colleague facilitates the exercise. Expense may however occur if an external facilitator is engaged.

USEFUL RESOURCE

● Blanchard & Alavi (2008) Asymmetry in the intensive care unit: Redressing imbalance and meeting the needs of family.

Processual interventions

These interventions aim to improve collaborative processes linked to the interprofessional work undertaken in a critical care unit. In general, these interventions aim to address practice-based issues, such as the use of checklists to help enhance interprofessional communication. Below is a range of interprofessional activities, which can help resolve processual issues.

Team policy

A team policy explicitly records the collective aims, roles and responsibilities of the team (Øvretveit, 1997). It also helps to ensure that a team has a formal document that provides members with details of how they operate. Each team policy should contain a number of key elements: an outline of the overall purpose of the team; information on team membership; clarification of individuals' roles within the team; details on the processes of teamwork; and shared targets/milestones.

FREQUENCY

On-going discussion between team members is required to ensure that their team policy is regularly updated and amended. For example, if a new member joins there may be a need to modify a previously agreed policy.

DURATION

A one-off staff meeting could be dedicated to developing the initial team policy, which could then be regularly reviewed and amended (if needed) in subsequent meetings.

COST

There should be no additional expense needed to implement team policy if a local colleague facilitates this activity. Again, as above, expense may however occur if an external facilitator is engaged to deliver this activity.

USEFUL RESOURCES

- www.who.int/cancer/modules/Team%20building.pdf (see Chapter 8).
- Øvretveit (1997) Planning and managing teams.

Team meetings

Designing team meetings that attempt to improve awareness and understanding of each other's roles, responsibilities and shared (patient/family-centred) goals can be a cost-effective approach to enhancing collaboration between clinical care staff as well as patients/families). Rather than introduce a new interprofessional meeting, it is recommended that an existing meeting is modified by dedicating a proportion of the meeting to discussing and collaboration and communication issues. Agreeing and then monitoring 'action plans' during meetings can help critical care staff implement follow-up actions to improve identified shortfalls.

FREQUENCY

Weekly or monthly – depending on which existing meeting can be used to focus on collaboration.

DURATION

Around 20 minutes of meeting time to review issues, plan and monitor any actions.

COST

Again, there should be no additional expense needed to implement discussions if an 'in-house' colleague facilitates the meeting. Expense may however occur if an external facilitator is engaged to deliver this activity.

USEFUL RESOURCES

- www.ihi.org/education/IHIOpenSchool/resources/Pages/Activities/Pozen Meetings.aspx
- https://blog.asana.com/2017/12/run-effective-meetings-agenda-tips/

Clinician–family meetings

Family members have reported that it is beneficial and comforting to organise regular clinician–family meetings with the specific goal of bringing families together as a group to discuss their critical care experiences. Such meetings in this context are adapted from stage one of the Family Intervention and Therapeutic Change Model developed by Robinson & Wright (1995). This model is founded on the principle that multiple realities exist for both family members and nurses, but that coming together as a group will foster the development of a relational, collaborative, consultative, and non-hierarchical relationship (Wright & Leahey, 2009). Regular meetings provide the space where families can have intentional interactions with their loved one's nurse in the hopes of developing deeper and more meaningful conversations. These meetings also serve as an acknowledgement to the family of the significance of having a loved one as critical care patient.

FREQUENCY

A regular monthly meeting with family members would ensure any on-going issues about involvement can be identified and addressed.

DURATION

Up to an hour meeting with family members arranged before or after a patient visit is recommended. Family members, if they would like, should be invited back to subsequent meetings

COST

Again, there should be no additional expense needed to implement reflexive discussions if an 'in-house' colleague facilitates the meeting. Expense may however occur if an external facilitator is engaged to deliver this activity. Refreshments should be provided.

USEFUL RESOURCE

- Nelms & Eggenberger (2010) The essence of the family critical illness experience and nurse family meetings.

Team checklists

Checklists are another cost-effective intervention that can help healthcare professionals explicitly concentrate on key care tasks they need to perform together. They can also help trigger communication and dialogue between members that can in turn improve their interprofessional relationships and relations with patients/family members. There are a number of checklists which have been created to support improved collaboration, such as SBAR (Situation-Background-Assessment-Recommendation) Tool.

FREQUENCY

Dependent on recommendations from individual checklists.

DURATION

Dependent on checklist activities.

COST

Checklists are generally free to download, though cost of implementation will vary depending on the toolkit activities.

USEFUL RESOURCES

- https://qi.elft.nhs.uk/resource/sbar-situation-background-assessment-recommendation/
- Thomas et al. (2009) The SBAR communication technique.

Care diaries and journals

A diary or journal is an on-going record of a patients' stay on a critical care unit. These documents can be kept by patients, family members, staff, managers and/or students. Photos, notes and letters can all be included. A diary/ journal can function as a therapeutic resource for the patient when recovering in the unit and also after discharge. These documents also have the potential to serve as a communication device between patients, families and critical care staff. The narratives they provide can offer staff with some very useful insights and understanding into the needs, values and perceptions held by the family. Critical care staff may also benefit from the positive acknowledgement and feedback the journal may contain.

FREQUENCY

Daily entries are recommended.

DURATION

Useful to have diary/journal records for a period of a week or so to identify regular issues, routines and practices.

COSTS

Notebooks and writing materials. Also, as this activity depends on the goodwill of individuals (e.g. patients, family members, students) to write these documents, a small gift of appreciation would be helpful.

USEFUL RESOURCES

- Egerod & Bagger (2010) Patients' experiences of intensive care diaries: A focus group study.

- Di Gangi et al. (2013) A narrative-based study on communication by family members in intensive care unit.

Toolkits

There are a growing number of toolkits available that can help improve identified difficulties with interprofessional collaboration as well as patient family involvement. These toolkits can be particularly helpful in providing a wide range of possible collaborative activities and quality improvement approaches. However, care is needed when using such toolkits to ensure their contents are applicable to the local critical care context they are being implemented within.

FREQUENCY
Dependent on the activities implemented from toolkit.

DURATION
Dependent on the activities implemented from toolkit.

COST
Usually free to download, though cost of activities will be dependent on the activities implemented from toolkit.

USEFUL RESOURCES
- www.ihi.org/resources/Pages/Tools/default.aspx
- www.education2practice.org/interprofessional-toolkit/

Redeveloping unit information

Pamphlets/leaflets with details about the environment, team members and formal and informal practices of a critical care unit are a simple, but helpful, intervention that can provide informational support for patients and family members. Having this information in a written format allows family members to refer back to the pamphlet at their leisure. It is best practice to write pamphlets in plain language in an accessible format that can be translated to suit diverse audiences. The content can include formal details about the hospital and the critical care unit, as well as informal practices or unspoken rules that are unique to the specific unit that the patient is currently in. To prevent misunderstandings between family members and staff, information should be reviewed and updated frequently.

FREQUENCY
On-going six-monthly reviews of unit pamphlets/leaflets are recommended.

DURATION

Time needed at staff meetings to review and revise unit materials – as required.

COST

Printing costs for new materials.

Organisational interventions

These interventions focus on improving collaboration and patient/family member involvement issues at an organisational level. These types of interventions may therefore be more complex to implement as they will involve agreement and support from more critical care stakeholders. Below is a range of interventions that can help address organisational issues.

Patient safety activities

The following activities can be used to prevent, detect and rectify interprofessional collaboration and communication errors in critical care setting. It consists of the following seven steps:

1 Identify a patient safety protocol to be used or develop a plan – it must be clear to everyone on the team what protocol or plan is being used.
2 Prioritise tasks for a patient – team members must understand how their individual tasks fit into the overall task.
3 Speak up – professionals must be prepared to speak up when patients are at risk. Team leaders must foster a climate which makes this possible.
4 Cross-monitor within the team – team members should watch each other for errors and problems. This should be seen not as criticism but as support for fellow members and an additional defence for patients.
5 Give and accept feedback – feedback should not be restricted to team leaders; any member should be able and prepared to give feedback to any other. But for this to be helpful, team members need to understand each other's roles.
6 Use closed loop communications – communications must be acknowledged and repeated by their recipients and even their senders. This provides an additional check and defence.
7 Back up other team members – members need to be aware of each other's actions and be ready to step in with support and assistance.

FREQUENCY

On-going – as organisational intervention this activity would become a part of a critical care unit's everyday patient safety practice.

DURATION

Once implementation agreed, daily.

COST

Mostly linked to implementation costs of intervention, which will be dependent on size of unit and number of staff.

USEFUL RESOURCE

- www.patientsafetyinstitute.ca/English/toolsResources/Pages/default.aspx

Clinical care pathways

Clinical care pathways are interventions in which the course of events and activities involved in a patient's care trajectory are specified within a certain time period. They aim to standardise processes related to the delivery of care and the clinical management of the patient. As such, pathways can be created or modified to ensure they have an explicit interprofessional collaboration and/or patient/family member-centred approach. They are particularly useful for relatively simple and predictable patient conditions. As a result, they may only be employed for a small fraction of the work undertaken by a critical care team.

FREQUENCY

On-going – as organisational intervention this activity would become a part of a critical care unit's everyday patient safety practice.

DURATION

Once implementation agreed, daily.

COST

Mostly linked to implementation costs of intervention, which will be dependent on size of unit and number of staff.

USEFUL RESOURCES

- www.rcn.org.uk/development/practice/perioperative_fasting/good_practice/service_improvement_tools/care_pathways
- www.icptoolkit.org/home.aspx

Re-organising care delivery

Changing the way care is organised within a critical care unit is one way to improve the quality of interprofessional collaboration and communication. Such interventions usually involve managers working with healthcare professionals to introduce new organisational policies or procedures which aim to, for instance, integrate the way care is delivered by different groups of professionals.

FREQUENCY

On-going – as organisational intervention this activity would become a part of a critical care unit's everyday interprofessional practice.

DURATION

Once implementation agreed this intervention is ongoing.

COST

Mostly linked to implementation costs of intervention, which will be dependent on size of unit and number of staff.

USEFUL RESOURCE

● www.atsjournals.org/doi/pdf/10.1164/rccm.200909-1441CP

Family member rounds

Rounds within critical care context can involve a range of different professions gathering together to discuss patients' clinical conditions. Typically, communication between family members and the healthcare team has not been considered a priority during these rounds. Indeed, some critical care units employ policies that restrict visiting hours when rounds are occurring. Family rounds can emphasise the patient and family member as the focal point of the discussion and encourage family member presence and participation. This configuration allows for a diversity of perspectives and gives the clinical staff an opportunity to answer any questions. Family members included in rounds report that they have a better understanding of patients' treatment plan as they have been involved in its development and daily refinement.

FREQUENCY

Weekly or monthly.

DURATION

One hour is recommended.

COST

Expenses should be paid for family members.

USEFUL RESOURCES

● Cypress (2012) Family presence on rounds: A systematic review of literature.

- Davidson (2013) Family presence on rounds in neonatal, pediatric and adult intensive care units.

Family support coordinator

Patients and family members in critical care often encounter a myriad of changing healthcare professionals, which can make continuity of care difficult to achieve. The purpose of a family support coordinator role is to provide family members with one point of contact whose responsibility it is to manage the flow of clinical information and to continually assess the unmet needs of the family. The family support coordinator can assist families in navigating the ICU setting by acting as a liaison between the family and medical team, clarifying complex medical information, and promoting family-centred decision-making. Having a family support coordinator on a unit can improve the degree to which the team members consider the needs of each family member.

FREQUENCY
Daily.

DURATION
Daily.

COST
Salary costs for new role.

USEFUL RESOURCE
- Shelton et al. (2010) The effect of a family support intervention on family satisfaction, length-of-stay, and cost of care in the intensive care unit.

Combining Interventions

One singular intervention may be ineffective in achieving sustained change in interprofessional collaboration and family involvement in the unit. Lasting change may be achieved through multi-faceted interventions that strengthen and reinforce positive practices. This could be done through implementing a combination of relational, processual, and organisational interventions presented above.[3]

Box 4.2 provides an example of how a relational, processual and organisational intervention can be employed in a complementary and effective fashion to tackle problems with interprofessional collaboration and patient/family member involvement.

BOX 4.2 Combining PROC interventions

INTERPROFESSIONAL COLLABORATION

Interventions to combine

1   relational: use of interprofessional team training sessions; *and*
2   processual: development of a shared team policy; *and*
3   organisational: introduction of a new care pathway to improve communication.

PATIENT/FAMILY INVOLVEMENT

Interventions to combine

1   relational: adoption of family assessment forms; *and*
2   processual: use of care diaries for patients/family members; *and*
3   organisational: introduction of family member rounds.

PART 3: EVALUATION

There is a clear need to evaluate any intervention(s) which are implemented to understand their impact on collaborative processes and/or patient/family member involvement. Efforts to gather this type of evidence can be extremely useful in having an empirical account of the effectiveness of any activity introduced into a critical care setting. As importantly, evaluation evidence can also generate insights into where interventions are failing, and so need amendment or modification. Chapter 5 provides more information on a range of different approaches, methods and tools that can be employed to generate a robust evaluation of all implemented intervention activities.

CONCLUDING COMMENTS

This chapter offered an account of a collaborative activity designed for critical care staff to identify a range of issues affecting collaboration and patient/family involvement in their critical care unit. Using the PROC framework the chapter also outlined a series of interventions aimed at improving identified shortfalls to help enhance the delivery of effective interprofessional patient/family-centred care.

NOTES

1   A mind map is a type of diagram often used for brainstorming. This type of map has a central problem or concept in the middle, with major associated concepts branching out.

2 For mind mapping with patients see: LaNoue et al. (2016) Concept mapping as a method to engage Patients in clinical quality improvement. *Annals of Family Medicine*; 14:370–376.

3 Interventions linked to context level factors are of course broader in scope, so their implementation depends on agencies outside the hospital (e.g. professional regulatory bodies) intervening in the form of regional and national policies that can affect local unit activities. As such, this type of intervention is not included in this workbook. Nevertheless, awareness of these factors is essential as they often frame relational-, processual- and organisational-level.

CHAPTER 5

Developing and undertaking
effective evaluation

....

INTRODUCTION

This chapter provides guidance on how to generate robust evidence to understand the effects of critical care interventions and activities created and implemented from the activities described in the previous chapters. The chapter is presented in the following way. First, some introductory information is offered about the nature and purpose of undertaking evaluation work. Second, a series of key methodological, ethical and practical issues are provided to help design and successfully evaluate interventions to improve collaboration between critical care staff, patients and families.

PART 1: WHAT IS EVALUATION?

Evaluation is a process of appraising activities in a formal and systematic way. A key purpose of evaluation is to make informed judgments about the usefulness of implemented interventions/activities. The purpose of an evaluation may be to provide formative information, summative information or both. Box 5.1 provides two examples of evaluation studies – one which employed formative approach and the other which employed a summative approach within a critical care context.

An evaluation that is undertaken early in the development of an intervention may be useful in understanding the influence of contextual factors as well as in providing information on how to improve the intervention (formative evaluation). In contrast, an evaluation undertaken once an intervention has been implemented typically focuses on its overall worth, e.g. effectiveness, efficiency, impact (summative evaluation).

BOX 5.1 Possible evaluation approaches

Formative evaluation: To generate an initial understanding of family member involvement in a critical care unit, this study employed a qualitative approach and gathered semi-structured interviews and observations. The findings suggested that family members particularly valued being involved in care decisions, however, at times, it was found that staff did not always include them. The findings from this formative evaluation were used to develop a series of seminars on how critical care staff could effectively engage family members in future decision-making.

Summative evaluation: This randomised control trial involved 20 critical care unit/homes (10 assigned to the experimental group and 10 to the control group) to examine the effects of monthly facilitated team rounds on the quality and quantity of care delivery. Participants included physicians, pharmacists, nurses and respiratory therapists. The trial found that the average number of drugs prescribed in the experimental units was the same before and after the intervention whereas the average number of drugs increased significantly in the control units. It was concluded that monthly team meetings improved prescribing of drugs in critical care.

Evaluation targets

Evaluations can also be grouped on the basis of their targets. An evaluation of an intervention may be focused on its inputs, processes, outcomes and/or impacts. Reeves et al. (2010) provide a series of evaluation questions in relation to these different targets (Table 5.1) which have been amended for a critical care context.

Types of evidence

When considering evaluation work, a key issue is whether *local evidence* or *generalisable evidence* is required. To understand the effects of collaborative critical care interventions across settings, generalisable evidence is required. Such evidence may also help to generate and test theories that offer insights into fundamental elements of collaboration between critical care staff, patients and their families.

Local evidence, available from a specific setting is always useful to gather. It can be used alongside other forms of evidence, to improve the organisation and delivery of local services. Local evidence is particularly useful to clinicians and managers responsible for care delivery in a particular clinical institution/unit. While generalisable evidence can assess the wider

TABLE 5.1 Evaluation questions for different intervention activities

Intervention focus	Areas to evaluate
Inputs	These may be training experiences, consultations and new critical care staff in order to achieve desired improvements in the organisation or delivery of care
Processes	Changes in work process, especially with regard to interactions among the critical care staff and patients/family members
Outcomes	These relate to the goals of the intervention and the extent to which the intervention has: • changed, increased or improved collaboration; • improved communication; • resulted in more inclusive consultation and decision-making between staff, patients and families.
Impacts	These relate to the goals of care delivered by critical care staff: • how and to what extent have changes been achieved in length of stay, health status changes, etc? • to what extent have critical care staff experiences improved, as measured by changes such as job satisfaction, work stress or staff turnover?

(Adapted from Reeves et al. 2010)

effects of an intervention, local evidence is needed for most other decisions about what actions should be taken.

All evaluations of interventions to improve collaboration between critical care staff, patients and families should aim to employ as rigorous evaluation methods as possible within resource constraints. Below we outline some key considerations when designing and implementing such evaluations.

PART 2: KEY EVALUATION ISSUES AND CONSIDERATIONS

In this section we outline a range of key elements that need to be considered when designing and implementing an evaluation.

Evaluation aim(s)

Formulating concise evaluation aim(s) is important because they will provide direction on which evaluation design is selected (below), which in turn will produce different results and conclusions. Examples of possible evaluation aims are:

- to determine whether an intervention improved family member involvement in the critical care unit;
- to study whether an intervention aimed at promoting improved collaboration between critical care staff led to improvements in the coordination of care.

Evaluation designs

There are a number of quantitative and qualitative evaluation designs available for use, as well as the option to combine approaches to produce a mixed-methods evaluation. In this section we review each of the main evaluation designs.

Quantitative designs

Below are the key quantitative designs that can be employed relatively inexpensively in a critical care setting when evaluating an intervention. In general, these types of design use a questionnaire or survey to obtain data from the participants of the intervention.

There are two main types of quantitative evaluation – descriptive and intervention studies. Descriptive studies (also called observational studies) use quantitative data to describe different phenomenon in different settings. Intervention studies are experiments in the sense that they focus on understanding what happens when an intervention is implemented.

DESCRIPTIVE STUDIES

Quantitative descriptive studies do not intervene in care delivery, nor do they implement any changes to the functioning of a particular unit. Instead, they aim to measure the effects/impact of interventions by looking at and comparing existing processes and outcomes. While these types of studies can be useful in generating a hypothesis that a particular intervention may result in improved outcomes, there is risk in using descriptive designs as the conclusions on the usefulness of activities that occur in a critical care setting. The problem is that such designs can generate confusion between cause and result. Confounding differences between individuals and/or units may prevent valid conclusions on effectiveness from being drawn. As a result, caution is needed in drawing conclusions on the effectiveness of intervention(s).

INTERVENTION STUDIES

Interventions can generate, effective, neutral or ineffective results. Empirical information on the effects of interventions is therefore needed to inform the allocation of resources for clinical activities and services. Below we outline a range of different quantitative intervention studies which can be employed.

Post-intervention study. This is the simplest type of design. It involves gathering data immediately after an intervention (e.g. staff training to improve family member involvement) has been implemented to gather an insight of the participants' perceptions about the effects of the intervention(s).

Before-and-after study. This design involves the collection of data before and after the intervention. This design helps detect changes resulting from an intervention more accurately as there is data collection at two points in time: before and after the intervention.

Interrupted times series study. This design aims to obtain a longitudinal account of the effects of an intervention over time. It uses different data collection points before and after an intervention to determine if it has an effect that is greater than any underlying trends. This design usually requires multiple time points (usually two to three) before the intervention to identify any underlying trends, and multiple points (usually two to three) afterwards to see if there is any change in the trend measured previously.

Qualitative designs

Below are some examples of qualitative designs, which can be employed relatively inexpensively. In general, these types of design gather observational, interview and/or documentary data from the participants of the intervention:

PHENOMENOLOGY

This form of inquiry brings individuals' perceptions of human experience with all types of phenomena. In a critical care context, phenomenology is an approach that allows for the exploration and description of phenomena important to staff, patients and their families through a small number of interviews with the intervention participants.

ETHNOGRAPHY

This type of design aims to study the interactions, behaviours and perceptions that can occur within a critical care unit. The central aim of ethnography is to provide an in-depth insight into people's views and actions, as well as the nature of the workspaces they inhabit, through the collection of observations and interviews. To keep costs down, it is encouraged that a rapid ethnographic approach is used – involving gathering data over a period of few days over a 2- to 3-week period.

ACTION RESEARCH

This type of design is a form of research that involves people in a process of change, which is based on professional and organisational action. It adopts a more collaborative approach than the designs described above, where the evaluators also work with intervention participants in processes of planning, implementing and evaluating change.

Mixed methods designs

If it is decided that a more comprehensive insight is needed, both quantitative and qualitative data should be gathered in a mixed-methods approach. This type of design aims to gather different types of quantitative and qualitative data (e.g. surveys, interviews, documents, observations) to provide a more detailed understanding of the processes and outcomes associated in an intervention. Comparing results between the different types of data can help generate more insightful findings of the effects of the intervention(s).

Ethical issues

Evaluating interprofessional collaboration and/or family involvement interventions inevitably requires ethical clearance. However, if your evaluation is to gain information for internal quality improvement purposes and will not be disseminated to external audiences, ethical approval may not be required. If you wish to disseminate your work further, it is recommended that ethical approval be obtained from all relevant research ethic boards.

Resources

Finding time and money for evaluating interventions can be difficult. Wherever possible one should consider where to secure funding for some or all stages of the evaluation process – formulation of evaluation aims, selection of designs, ethical approval, data collection, data analysis and dissemination of results.

Use of evaluation tools

There are numerous interprofessional and collaborative pre-validated tools that can be used to gather data during an evaluation. One particularly useful online resource to access has been created by the US National Center for Interprofessional Practice and Education which has collated a number of measurement tools and other resources to support interprofessional evaluation:
https://nexusipe.org/advancing/assessment-evaluation-start

Stakeholder involvement

Evaluation often involves a wide range of stakeholders with an interest in the conduct and findings of the evaluation (e.g. critical care staff, managers, patients, family members). Evaluation aims and methods may need to be negotiated with these groups, therefore it is important to identify these stakeholder groups and approach them for input/feedback on the design and implementation of an evaluation. They can also be helpful with dissemination of evaluation results – see below.

Change

Change is a constant within a critical care setting. As a result, any evaluation can be difficult to control, as both context and intervention may be changing as the evaluation progresses. Evaluations are also often limited by a range of local changes, such as time and funding constraints, or the loss of local intervention champion(s), which can undermine ongoing evaluation work.

Employing an internal or external evaluator

Similar to the issues mentioned in Chapter 1, an 'insider' evaluator can benefit from extensive knowledge of the history and context of a study setting, but that can make it difficult to stand back from the data and interpret it in a neutral manner. In contrast, external evaluators may find it easier to view their work from a more neutral viewpoint. This neutrality is also helpful for eliciting more candid data from participants. However, they often have to spend time, and money developing an in-depth understanding of contextual issues.

Reactivity

Also known as The Hawthorne Effect, reactivity refers to a phenomenon where the presence of the evaluator positively changes research participants' behaviour. Assessing the level of reactivity on an evaluation is difficult, but you need to be aware of its presence and its possible effects. Overtime, reactivity issues diminish, as individuals cannot usually alter their behaviour for long due to managing busy clinical workloads.

Dissemination

Disseminating the results from an evaluation is an important part of the process. It provides participants, managers, employers, funders, etc. with important information about the success (or not) of intervention(s). There are a number of different routes of dissemination to consider, including:

- Local meetings: useful for updating colleagues, clinical managers and family members about the evaluation work.
- National or international conferences or meetings (posters, papers): these are useful places to discuss early work to elicit feedback on processes and/or outcomes.

- Short reports in professional journals: these are particularly useful for describing work in progress and/or directing readers to a more lengthy report.
- Peer-reviewed papers: these can provide more information on the intervention and evaluation, usually for an academic audience.
- Websites/blogs/social media – these applications can provide rapid, easily updated, low-cost access to evaluation information. Feedback can also be obtained from those who use the site.

Evaluation checklist

Table 5.2 provides a simple checklist to use to help when both designing and then implementing an evaluation of a critical care intervention to improve collaboration between staff, patients and families.

Concluding comments

This chapter aimed to provide advice on how to design and implement evaluation studies to understand the effects of critical care interventions and activities described in previous chapters. The evaluation information presented in this chapter related to methodological, ethical and practical issues aimed to ensure that any evaluation work has been designed to produce a high-quality study which can be successfully implemented across critical care settings.

TABLE 5.2 An evaluation checklist

Key questions	Responses
What critical care intervention(s) are to be evaluated and what are our evaluation question(s)?	1.
What evaluation design will be employed?	2.
Who will be undertaking the evaluation?	3.
What resources are available for the use of the evaluation?	4.
Have we considered all ethical dimensions? (If needed, have we secured ethical approval?)	5.
How will we deal with bias (e.g. reactivity) in our evaluation?	6.
How have we involved key stakeholders in our evaluation?	7.
What evaluation tools are we going to use?	8.
What are the costs to undertake the evaluation?	9.
What is our dissemination plan?	10.

(Adapted from Reeves et al. 2015b)

CHAPTER 6

Concluding comments

....

This workbook aimed to offer a series of robust and developed assessment, implementation and evaluation activities designed to improve collaboration between critical care professionals, patients and family members. As previously noted, materials for this workbook were empirically developed from qualitative data generated from a study of different ICUs. Uniquely, this workbook offered activities based on data that examined the daily working practices of these ICUs.

While the initial focus of the data for the activities were gathered in North America, we have attempted to develop a set of activities which have resonance with a wider number of national contexts such as Australia, Brazil, Denmark, Germany, Japan, South Africa, Sweden and the UK and the different professional groups (e.g. physicians, nurses, respiratory therapists, pharmacists, social workers) who work in critical care settings in these countries.

Overall, our aim was that this workbook would help readers (from a number of backgrounds, e.g. professionals, family members, managers, policy makers, researchers, educators, students) understanding of key issues linked to collaboration between critical care staff, patients and families. In doing so, a central element for the book has been the PROC framework (Figure 0.1) developed to help understand the nature of interprofessional teamwork. This framework has usefully provided a set of conceptual lenses to help view the varying different factors related to collaboration in a critical care setting.

Throughout the book, we have paid particular attention to implementation issues, regularly providing ideas on how, where and when (with ideas on possible costs) to implement intervention and evaluation activities. For example, we have noted how engagement with patient safety colleagues will be helpful in implementation. Also, how the tools presented in this workbook can be easily incorporated with existing unit activities.

Another core element of the book has been our stress on considering local context to help understand the nature of local practices in order to tailor interventions that are impactful. This focus on context can be found in our repeated calls for careful assessment of collaboration and family/patient involvement issues before designing and implementing an intervention.

Finally, we have been keen to stress the need for robust evaluation. Without generating good quality evidence one cannot know how effective (or ineffective) any implemented activity designed to improve collaboration between critical care staff, patients and family members. As such, intervention should never occur without evaluation.

We hope that the assessment, intervention and evaluation activities described in this workbook will be of use to critical care colleagues to identify and improve any shortfalls or deficiencies they identify with interprofessional collaboration and/or patient/family member involvement. As stressed throughout the book, these activities have all been designed to be practical and easy to implement across different critical care settings. We would be delighted to hear any comments (positive or negative) from colleagues on their experiences of using any of the activities. Our plan is to use any feedback received to further develop/fine tune the quality of the assessment, intervention and evaluation activities presented in previous chapters.

APPENDIX 1

Background context

....

This workbook is based on a two-year, multi-sited ethnographic study entitled, *Understanding the nature of team-based care and patient and family involvement in intensive care settings: a multi-site study*. This study had three major objectives: to explore interprofessional care and family involvement in North America; to develop an empirically-based tool to assess the quality of team-based care and patient and family involvement; and to develop a package of interventions to strengthen team-based care and patient and family involvement.

STUDY HIGHLIGHTS
- Eight intensive care units across North America.
- Over 1,000 hours of observation of interprofessional work, communication, and collaboration, as well as interactions between healthcare providers and patient family members.
- Eighty clinician interviews and thirty-seven patient and family member interviews.

SELECTED PUBLICATIONS
For those interested in reading more about this study see (in chronological order):

Reeves, S., Paradis, E., Leslie, M., Kitto, S., Aboumatar, H., Gropper M. (2013) Understanding the nature of interprofessional collaboration and patient family involvement in intensive care settings: a study protocol. *ICU Director*. http://icu.sagepub.com/content/4/5/242
Paradis, E., Reeves, S., Leslie, M., Aboumatar, H., Chesluk, B., Clark, P., et al. (2014) Exploring the nature of interprofessional collaboration and family member

involvement in an intensive care context. *Journal of Interprofessional Care*; 28:74–75.

Alexanian, J., Kitto, S., Rak, K., Reeves, S. (2015) Beyond the team: understanding interprofessional work in two North American ICUs. *Critical Care Medicine*; 43(9):1880–1886.

Reeves, S., McMillan, S., Kachan, N., Paradis, E., Leslie, M., Kitto, S. (2015) Interprofessional collaboration and family member involvement in intensive care units: emerging themes from a multi-sited ethnography. *Journal of Interprofessional Care*; 29(3):230–237.

Reeves, S., Kitto, S., Alexanian, J., Grant, R. (2016) *Enhancing interprofessional collaboration in the intensive care unit: a toolkit.* Available at: https://nexusipe.org/informing/resource-center/eic-icu-toolkit-enhancing-interprofessional-collaboration-intensive-care.

Olding, M., McMillan, S., Reeves, S., Schmitt, M., Puntillo, K., Kitto, S. (2016) Patient and family involvement in adult critical and intensive care settings: a scoping review. *Health Expectations*; 19:1183–1202.

Kendall-Gallagher, D., Reeves, S., Alexanian, J., Kitto, S. (2016) A nursing perspective of interprofessional work in critical care: a secondary analysis. *Journal of Critical Care*; 38:20–26.

Goldman, J., Kitto, S., Reeves, S. (2018) Examining the implementation of collaborative competencies in a critical care setting: key challenges for enacting competency-based education. *Journal of Interprofessional Care*. DOI:10.1080/1356 1820.2017.1401987.

Combining intervention approaches

....

As noted earlier in this book, the ideas, activities and tools presented in this workbook can be used collectively, as stand-alone activities, or can be incorporated into an existing interprofessional team program such as the very well-known CUSP (Comprehensive Unit Based Safety Program).[1] CUSP is ideal for this purpose, not only because it provides a framework for organisational change, which is applied to the specific concerns of a critical care unit (as identified by frontline staff), but also because it recognises the importance of cultural factors in the delivery of care. In order to enhance the CUSP process of adaptation to cultural context, we recognised the potential value of incorporating the activities described in this workbook to CUSP. Below we have indicated the synergy between these complementary approaches (additions are presented in *italics*).

PRE-CUSP
- Obtain leadership support
- Assemble a safety team (IP team, plus senior executive)
- Assess unit safety culture (survey)

CUSP
- Educate staff on science of safety

  - Science of safety presentation (small groups) and online training

- Identify defects

  - Staff safety assessment form

- *Defining and improving patient and family involvement* (see Chapter 3)
- *Identifying and addressing issues that affect care delivery* (see Chapter 4)
- Collate responses and consider existing data

● Senior executive partnership

- Identify senior executive
- Unit safety team meets and orients
- Monthly rounds
- Safety rounds
- Identify and manage improvement projects

● Learning from defects

- Identify safety defect
- Complete case summary

● Teamwork tools

- Implement Multidisciplinary Rounds with Daily Goals
- Implement Structured Huddles
- Learn from one defect on the unit using tools from the CUSP toolkit

● Enable culture conducive to safety improvements

- Morning briefing tool
- Shadowing professional tool

● Daily goals tool

- Defining and improving interprofessional collaboration (see Chapter 2).

NOTE
1 See: www.ahrq.gov/professionals/quality-patient-safety/cusp/index.html

Advice for interviewing critical care staff

....

This appendix provides further advice on gathering the interview data on interprofessional collaboration as described in Chapter 2.

ETHICS

Ethical approval may not be required if your interviews are being conducted to only gain information for internal purposes (e.g. quality improvement). However, your institution may require approval from a Research Ethics Committee if you intend to publish your findings. It is therefore best to consult with your institutional policies before setting up interviews.

RECRUITMENT

- Seek out healthcare professionals from a variety of professional backgrounds.
- Keep in mind that clinicians have patient care responsibilities.
- Stress what is unique about this interview – they get to talk about their experience.

SPACE

Ensure you have a private room booked for the interview. Set the room up beforehand if you can (e.g. appropriate number of chairs). Make sure the interviewee knows how to get there.

WHAT TO BRING

Interview script, pen, paper, consent form (if applicable), recorder with extra batteries (if recording the interview)

CONDUCTING INTERVIEWS

- Use open body language and active listening skills. Paraphrase their answers to show you're listening and to confirm that you've understood what they are saying.
- Resist the urge to fill any silences and pauses.
- Try to avoid reading directly off the interview script if possible, and really listen to their answers. You may find that the questions come naturally if you're listening.

Advice for gathering observational data

....

This appendix provides further advice on gathering the observational data on interprofessional collaboration as described in Chapter 2.

ETHICS

Ethical approval may not be required if your observations are being gathered to only gain information for internal purposes (e.g. quality improvement). However, your institution may require approval from a Research Ethics Committee if you intend to publish your findings. It is therefore best to consult with your institutional policies before beginning data collection.

WHAT TO BRING

Writing utensils, notebook, consent forms (if applicable)

WHAT TO DO

- Take field notes regularly.
- Write up field notes promptly.
- Try to be inconspicuous so you don't intimidate staff or family members. At times you may want to retreat to a quiet area to write down your notes.
- Analyse your notes frequently. Are there any emerging findings you want to observe further? Are you missing anything substantial, such as night shifts?

FIELD NOTE EXAMPLE

Below is an example of a real field note from the study that informed this toolkit. Key points for consideration are listed in the right column.

Field note	Key points
3:25pm RN1 walks into the pnt2's room, who is unresponsive, checks the monitors by the bedside and then begins talking to the two visitors. RN1 explains that visitor policy is 2 at a time and asks them to remind their family members of the policy. The pnt2 visitors speak amongst themselves in their native language (they speak Farsi and appear confused at the information they just received). RN1 looks at me and shrugs her shoulders (she seems to be indicating that she is trying her best to communicate). 3:35pm RN2 (a senior nurse) walks by, pauses at the entrance way briefly and comes and stands beside RN1; they smile at each other and address each other by first name. RN1 says to RN2 that she is unsure of how much the visitors understand. RN2 says directly to the visitors "So, so far just antibiotics. Antibiotic. We might use a mask." One of the visitors replies, in broken English, "Ok. More oxygen." RN1 and RN2 both nod and confirm that is the plan. RN1 and RN2 move closer	• Periodically noting the time to give the reader a better sense of the events. • Use pseudonyms, such as RN1, to protect anonymity. • Include your impressions and add information in brackets. • Make note when your presence as an observer is acknowledged. • Make note of intraprofessional interactions, here the RN2 sees that RN1 may be having a communication problem and comes to help and offer support without being asked. They work together to speak with the family and then discuss the care plan. • Use direct quotes when you can jot them down. • Note impressions if you are uncertain. • Make note of interpersonal interactions, here a resident and nurse coordinate their care efforts and the resident offers assistance by communicating with the family. • How medical information is communicated and received is just as important as the medical information itself.

continued . . .

Continued

Field note	Key points
to the doorway and a side conversation (inaudible but their gestures to the patient file RN1 is holding, it appears to be about the care plan). 3:45pm Res5 approaches and says, to RN1 "I speak Farsi." And RN1 says, "Oh good!" (she is visibly relieved). RN1 updates RN15 that the visitors know about the medications being administered and that she gave the antibiotics one hour ago. RN2 raises a medical question about the timing of medications: "I noticed that [technical information about IV] but I was wondering if maybe [technical issue, citing evidence]. But maybe that's been considered already?" Res5 looks at patient as RN2 is talking and does not make eye contact, when she is finished he gestures to see the patient file.	

Guidance for facilitating the initial staff workshop

....

This appendix provides facilitation guidance to support the initial workshop described in Chapter 2. Also see Appendix 9 for more general suggestions about facilitation.

FACILITATION TIPS

When choosing a facilitator, possibilities include:

- experienced critical care professional;
- representative from the hospital's patient safety or quality improvement unit;
- representative from hospital's in-service training department.

MATERIALS

Writing instruments, sticky notes, chart paper

TIME

1.5 to 3 hours

SUGGESTED PROCESS FOR WORKSHOP FACILITATION

1 Welcome the staff.
2 Introduce yourself and your role in this initiative.
3 Describe the purpose of the workshop:

- To share the findings of the interviews and observations, and explore different perceptions of interprofessional communication/interactions within their critical care unit.

4 Review the agenda with the participants:

- Discuss the types of health professions we work with and how we work together.
- Explore the flow of interprofessional communication and interaction in our ICU.
- Questions for reflection.

5 Give each participant pens/markers, a stack of blank card and a large sheet of paper. If you have a large group, have everyone split into inter-professional groups of approximately five people.

6 Defining the healthcare professionals:

- Ask the participants to use the cards provided to write down all the healthcare professionals that work in the ICU.
- Ask participants to explain and compare their lists.

7 Defining interprofessional dynamics:

- Ask the participants to create a pile from the list of healthcare professionals that represents staff in their unit that work together.
- Ask participants to explain how they made their selections. Who did you include? Who did you leave out?

8 Share the findings from observations and interviews:

- Share examples from the observations and interviews.
- Ask participants how these examples and findings resonate with their experience.

9 Creating an interaction chart:

- Ask the participants to revisit their cards. Has their perception changed at all since hearing the results of the interviews and observations? How, or why not?
- Ask the participants to arrange the cards to depict flows of communication and interaction within their ICU. Encourage them to arrange the cards on top of the blank sheet and use markers to signify flows of information and add in any additional information about interactions.
- Facilitate a discussion on how the participants have arranged their interaction charts.

10 Reflection and discussion:

- Ask the participants to reflect and share what they think the activity says about the way different professionals in their unit work together.
- Did anything surprise them?
- What changes (if any) can they make to how they work with other healthcare professionals?

Guidance for facilitating the family involvement workshop

....

This appendix aims to provide facilitation guidance to support the family involvement workshop described in Chapter 3. Also see Appendix 9 for more general suggestions about facilitation.

FACILITATING TIPS
When choosing a facilitator, there are a number of possibilities, including:

- A staff member or external resource person can serve as a facilitator.
- If using in conjunction with CUSP, a member of the CUSP "safety team" can serve as a facilitator.
- It may also be beneficial to have the workshop co-facilitated by a patient/family rep if there is one available at your institution.

MATERIALS
Writing instruments, paper, sticky notes (two colours), previously collected *Family Involvement Records*.

TIME
45 to 60 minutes.

SUGGESTED PROCESS FOR WORKSHOP FACILITATION
1 Welcome the staff.
2 Introduce yourself and your role in this initiative.

3 Describe the purpose of the workshop:

- To explore different perceptions of family involvement, and discuss how family involvement can be enhanced in your unit.

4 Review the agenda with the participants:

- Complete the "Reflection on Family Involvement in the Delivery of Care" card.
- Review the *Family Involvement Records*.
- Review the *Healthcare Professional Reflection Cards*.
- Questions for reflection.

5 Activity 1: "Reflection on Family Involvement in the Delivery of Care" card

- Distribute a piece of paper to each participant.
- Ask participants to write down what role they see for family in the delivery of care. Ask them to keep their reflections anonymous.
- Once the participants are done writing, collect the cards. Inform the participants that you will be coming back to these cards closer to the end of the session.

6 Activity 2: Reviewing completed Family Involvement Records

- Divide everyone into groups and distribute the *Family Involvement Records*. Allow the groups time to review the records.
- Ask participants to describe what emerging understanding they see. Have the participants write these key findings onto sticky notes.
- Bring the whole group together to arrange similar findings into themes by grouping similar sticky notes on the wall.
- Ask participants how these findings resonate with their experiences. What impact do these kinds of involvements have on their work?

7 Activity 3: Reviewing Healthcare Professional Reflection Cards

- Distribute the *Healthcare Professional Reflection Cards* and sticky notes (colour not used in Activity 2) to the groups. Allow the groups time to review their cards.
- Ask participants to describe what emerging understanding they see. Have the participants write these key findings onto sticky notes.
- Bring the whole group together to arrange similar findings into themes by grouping similar sticky notes on the wall. Some themes may be the same as those identified in Activity 2, or there may be new themes.
- Ask the participants to reflect and share what they think the activity tells us about the way their unit deals with family involvement.

- Are there differences between how family members describe their involvement and what healthcare professionals' understanding is?
- What surprises you?
- What changes (if any) can you make in your clinical practice to facilitate family involvement?

Guidance for facilitating the collaborative critical care workshop

....

This appendix aims to provide facilitation guidance to support the collaborative critical care workshop described in Chapter 4. Also see Appendix 9 for more general suggestions about facilitation.

WORKSHOP PREPARATION

It is recommended that the facilitator consult the checklists in Appendix 8 before meeting with the group. Previous reflection on some of the underlying issues impacting interprofessional teamwork will allow for enhanced workshop facilitation.

FACILITATING TIPS

When choosing a facilitator, a member of the CUSP "safety team" (see Appendix 1) or, ideally, an experienced healthcare professional should lead the session.

MATERIALS

Different coloured pens/markers, chart paper

TIME

1.5 hours

SUGGESTED PROCESS

1 Welcome the staff.
2 Introduce yourself and your role in this initiative.

3 Describe the purpose of the workshop:

- To identify an interprofessional/patient/family problem on the unit and take the first steps towards resolving it.

4 Review the agenda with the participants:

- Identification of issues impacting collaboration and/or patient care on the unit.
- Creation of a mind map through collaborative brainstorming to explore what is contributing to the problem.
- Examine the connections between these factors.
- Discuss where an intervention would be most effective.
- Questions for reflection.

5 Ask the participants to consider the following questions:

- What are some issues that are impacting teamwork and/or patient care on our unit?
- Why might these issues exist?

6 Invite the participants to share some of the concerns they have identified, and make a list on the chart paper.

7 Ask the participants to select the issue that they believe is most important to focus on for the rest of the session. Depending on the size of the group, you may be able to split everyone into two groups to explore two issues.

8 Collaborative brainstorming:

- Write the identified problem into the middle of the mind map.
- Ask the participants to consider what forces may be facilitating or restraining the problem.
- Record participants' ideas on the mind map, organised by the PROC framework – processual, relational, organisational, and contextual.

9 Making connections:

- Ask the participants if they see any connections between the factors listed on the mind map.
- Ask the participants who is involved in the issue and the major factors contributing to it. Who should the intervention target – frontline staff, team processes, organisation of care?

10 Reflection and discussion:

- How do these issues impact your clinical practice?
- How do these issues impact patients and families?

Checklists for identifying interprofessional and patient/family issues

....

This appendix contains four checklists designed to be used during the collaborative critical care activity.

The factors identified in the checklists below were key factors identified
in our data. Informed by the PROC framework, these findings were further
examined in relation to the wider literature on interprofessional work in
critical care in order to distil key issues that could be used to help individual
units assess their own unit's clinical context. This information was streamlined
into these checklists to provide facilitators with a straightforward and tangible
way to begin assessing their unit's interprofessional issues.

Below are two real-life examples (from the ICU study data) of how a
clinician's perspectives can be interpreted by use of the PROC framework.
In the first quote, a nurse describes a *processual factor*:

> It depends on how busy the day is. Usually what happens is if you
> notice your patient needs something, certain things you will go ahead
> and do because they don't really require authorization or you wait until
> rounds to bring it up. But other things you'll just go to the doctor
> and speak to them for a moment and quickly say what the problem
> is and what you think you need. In most cases, they'll say 'yes, go
> ahead and do that'. It's more so just a formality just getting that
> approval but that's typically how things can happen.

In the following quote, a physician describes some *organisational factors*
that impact interprofessional teamwork and patient care:

So, for example, when there are conflicts about whether patients should be aggressively resuscitated when, medically, it's very difficult to foresee any good outcomes for them, other hospitals might have a culture saying we are not going to do this. This is not medically indicated and we're willing to stand on this line and fight it all the way to the Supreme Court, for example, versus, [here], what I've been told at least, is don't even bother. The culture here is to do whatever the family says, and not fight those fights, because they don't think it's worthwhile. That's been my experience, as well. If you look at our list, almost all of our patients are for resuscitation, even if they have two metastatic cancers, and obviously, no real chance of a great outcome, the decision has been made to respect the family's choice and the patient's choice, and not add extra stress and just go with it. And, as a trainee who rotates through, you go with the flow of the culture, you don't try to change it.

CHECKLIST 1 Processual factors				
Interprofessional factors				
Factor	**Example**	**How manifested on the unit?**	**What are the risks?**	**Possible solutions**
Time/space	*A physician changes a patient care plan in the electronic record during nurse handover*			
Routines/ rituals	*Rounds geared to teaching limit opportunity for interprofessional interactions*			
Information technology	*Physicians' use of workstations on wheels during rounds affects face to face com- munication*			

continued . . .

CHECKLIST 1 Continued				
Interprofessional factors				
Factor	**Example**	**How manifested on the unit?**	**What are the risks?**	**Possible solutions**
Unpredict-ability	*Pharmacist and nurse talk about medication management plan in antici-pation of an unpredictable patient event*			
Urgency	*An emergency medical procedure is prioritised over inter-professional communication needs*			
Complexity	*A respiratory therapist and physician have different perspectives on patient care plan in a com-plex patient*			
Other factors (to be added)				
Patient/family factors				
Physical environment	*Technologically invasive landscape of ICU can inhibit or intimidate family member involvement*			

continued . . .

CHECKLIST 1 Continued				
Interprofessional factors				
Factor	**Example**	**How manifested on the unit?**	**What are the risks?**	**Possible solutions**
Complexity	*Multiple specialists involved in the care of a patient can be confusing for patient's family members*			
Routines/ rituals	*Rounds where staff discuss care plans can feel intimidating and/or exclusionary to family members*			
Other factors (to be added)				

CHECKLIST 2 Relational factors				
Interprofessional factors				
Factor	**Example**	**How manifested on the unit?**	**What are the risks?**	**Possible solutions**
Professional power	*Physician decision to discharge a patient is in tension with a nurse's perspective that patient is not suitable for discharge*			

continued . . .

CHECKLIST 2 Continued

Interprofessional factors

Factor	Example	How manifested on the unit?	What are the risks?	Possible solutions
Hierarchy	*A nurse is not comfortable questioning a medication decision by a physician*			
Socialisation	*A respiratory therapist and physician have different perspectives on patient readiness for extubation*			
Team composition	*The presence of healthcare professionals such as social workers and pharmacists on a unit create opportunities for teamwork*			
Team roles	*A speech language pathologist's role is not understood by other staff, is rarely included in discussion*			

continued . . .

CHECKLIST 2 Continued				
Interprofessional factors				
Factor	**Example**	**How manifested on the unit?**	**What are the risks?**	**Possible solutions**
Team processes	*Physicians and nurses working together over time develop trust and respect in contrast to temporary workers*			
Other factors (to be added)				
Patient/family factors				
Team roles	*The boundaries of professional roles may be unclear to patient's family members*			
Trust and respect	*Trust and respect between staff and patient's family members can be fostered and inhibited by previously shared interactions*			
Other factors (to be added)				

CHECKLIST 3 Organisational factors				
Interprofessional factors				
Factor	**Example**	**How manifested on the unit?**	**What are the risks?**	**Possible solutions**
Organisational support	*The critical care management agrees to organise regular inter-professional rounds*			
Professional representation	*Clinical leaders promote linkages across professional groups*			
Fear of litigation	*Concerns of litigation related to comprises in patient safety undermine interprofes-sional decision-making*			
Other factors (to be added)				
Patient/family factors				
Fear of litigation	*Communication between staff and family members affected by fear of litigation related to criticism from patient's relatives*			

continued . . .

CHECKLIST 3 Continued				
Interprofessional factors				
Factor	**Example**	**How manifested on the unit?**	**What are the risks?**	**Possible solutions**
Unit specific policies	*Unit policies relating to visiting hours not apparent to family members or not enforced uniformly by staff*			
Other factors (to be added)				

CHECKLIST 4 Contextual factors				
Interprofessional factors				
Factor	**Example**	**How manifested on the unit?**	**What are the risks?**	**Possible solutions**
Culture	*Sub-groups of professional and inter-professional teams impede unit teamwork*			
Diversity	*Diversity in teams with greater amounts of views and approaches can challenge teamwork*			
Gender	*Patriarchal arrangements reproduced in interprofes-sional teams*			

continued . . .

CHECKLIST 4 Continued

Interprofessional factors

Factor	Example	How manifested on the unit?	What are the risks?	Possible solutions
Political will	*Policies promoting interprofessional teamwork create a climate for teamwork*			
Economics	*Managerial imperatives concerning patient flow can affect different professionals' perspectives about patient readiness for discharge creating communication challenges*			
Other factors (to be added)				
Patient/family factors				
Diversity	*Cultural differences can lead to misunderstandings between staff and patient's family members*			

continued . . .

CHECKLIST 4 Continued

Interprofessional factors

Factor	Example	How manifested on the unit?	What are the risks?	Possible solutions
Gender	*Different cultural rules related to gender can create a disconnect between staff and family members*			
Political will	*Policies promoting patient and family-centred care can lead to tensions between staff and family members*			
Economics	*Socioeconomic factors may prevent family members from being consistently present on the unit so less available for interactions with staff*			
Other factors (to be added)				

General facilitation guidance

....

General facilitation guidance is presented below to complement and support the specific facilitation guidance presented in Appendices 5, 6, and 7.

BEFORE A WORKSHOP

Time

Consider the amount of time the group can feasibly spend together. Depending on the group and workshop, you may need to decrease the amount of time spent in each workshop. Some ideas for decreasing workshop time include:

- Use dedicated time where you can, such as in-service training sessions and bi/monthly meetings.
- Split up the workshop into two shorter sessions.
- Ask participants to complete some of the more self-reflective work ahead of time. Make sure participants are given ample notice and clear instructions for any pre-work.
- Consider whether there are any learning activities that can be 'flipped', i.e. where participants could be sent materials to review/read ahead of the workshop, ensuring more time to active learning during the workshop.

Space

Make sure the room you are using for the workshop is appropriate for the workshop. Some things to consider:

- Is it an appropriate size for the number of people?
- Does the space work for the kind of activities you are going to be doing?
- If any of the participants have patient care responsibilities (e.g. on-call), is the space close to the unit?

Materials

Make sure you have all of the materials you will need, such as paper, markers, and any audio-visual equipment you wish to use. Ensure all materials are working beforehand.

Facilitator

Consider who will be leading the workshop, and the implications this could have on the success of the workshop. For example, would staff be willing to share examples of controversial behaviours and views if the ICU manager is in the room? Could there be interprofessional conflict if the workshop is led by a physician? A nurse? Consider others who can add richness to the workshop. For example, it would be advantageous to involve a family member representative. From an interprofessional standpoint, it would also be beneficial to have various professions involved in the planning and delivery of the workshops.[1]

DURING A WORKSHOP

Time management

Keep track of time during the workshop. For group activities, tell participants how long they will have to complete the activities, and give them warning before moving on to the next item.

Active listening

Use active listening skills to show participants that you are listening and to ensure you understand their message. Repeat back what participants are saying by paraphrasing, and request clarification and confirmation as necessary.

Evaluation

Remember to distribute your evaluation forms. The feedback received here can be useful in planning future workshops. Additionally, some participants may feel more comfortable sharing some of their ideas anonymously. If you are rushed for time, you can also use an online survey tool. See Appendix 10 for an example of an evaluation sheet which could be employed.

AFTER A WORKSHOP

Evaluation

Remember to collect your evaluation forms. If you used an electronic format, send out a follow-up email a few days to a week after the evaluation form/survey was sent out. Remind the participants to complete the evaluation form, and thank them for their participation.

Record keeping
Make sure you keep a record of the ideas and thoughts shared during the workshop before disposing of any workshop material.

Clean up
Make sure you leave the room in the condition you found it.

NOTE
1. Van Hoof et al. (2015) Society for Academic Continuing Medical Education intervention guideline series: Interprofessional Education. *Journal of Continuing Education for the Health Professions*; 35: S60–S64.

Possible evaluation form

....

Below is an evaluation form which could be used to provide immediate feedback on any of the workshop activities described in Chapters 2, 3, and 4.

Thank you for attending the XXX activity. Please complete this evaluation form and submit it to the facilitator.

Statement	5 Excellent	4 Above average	3 Average	2 Below average	1 Poor
Please rate your overall satisfaction with the workshop with respect to the following:					
Overall evaluation of the workshop					
How useful is the workshop to you professionally?					
How useful is the workshop to you personally?					
Did the workshop meet your expectations?					
Comments:					

continued . . .

Continued					
Activities					
How effective was your group in working together during the activities?					
Usefulness of the activities to achieving workshop goals					
Comments:					
What other issues would you like to see addressed in the unit?					
General recommendations or comments:					

Online resources

....

In this appendix we provide information on organisations which promote interprofessional collaboration and family-centred care, and their related websites.

AMERICAN INTERPROFESSIONAL HEALTH COLLABORATIVE (AIHC)

The AIHC offers a venue for health and social professions based in the USA to share information, mentor and support one another as they provide the leadership to influence system change with the implementation of interprofessional education and practice at their individual institutions and organisations.

Website: https://aihc-us.org/

AUSTRALASIAN INTERPROFESSIONAL PRACTICE AND EDUCATION NETWORK (AIPPEN)

AIPPEN aims to provide a forum for the sharing of information, networks and experiences in the area of interprofessional practice and education in health and social care contexts across Australia and New Zealand.

Website: www.aippen.net/

CANADIAN INTERPROFESSIONAL HEALTH COLLABORATIVE (CIHC)

The CIHC is a Canadian national organisation that provides health providers, teams, and organisations with the resources and tools needed to apply an interprofessional, patient-centred, and collaborative approach to healthcare. CIHC's core activities are designed to make them the key resource for these organisations when they require expert advice, knowledge, or information on interprofessional collaboration.

Website: www.cihc.ca

CENTRE FOR THE ADVANCEMENT OF INTERPROFESSIONAL EDUCATION (CAIPE)

Founded in 1987, CAIPE is dedicated to the promotion and development of interprofessional education with and through its individual and corporate members, in collaboration with likeminded organisations in the UK and overseas. It provides information and advice through its website, bulletins, papers and outlets provided by others, and has a close association with the *Journal of Interprofessional Care*. CAIPE also delivers workshops which facilitate development in IPE and foster exchange and mutual support between members and others.

Website: www.caipe.org.uk

EUROPEAN INTERPROFESSIONAL EDUCATION NETWORK (EIPEN)

European Interprofessional Education Network (EIPEN) aims to establish a sustainable inclusive network of people and organisations in partner countries to share and develop effective interprofessional learning and teaching for improving collaborative practice and multi-agency working in health and social care. EIPEN has two interlinked aims: to develop a transnational network of universities and employers in the six participating countries and to promote good practices in interprofessional learning and teaching (IPE) in health and social care.

Website: www.eipen.org

INSTITUTE FOR HEALTHCARE IMPROVEMENT

The Institute for Healthcare Improvement (IHI) aims to help build the will for change, cultivating concepts for improvement, and helping professions and managers implement ideas into action. The IHI also works to change the skills, attitudes, and knowledge of the health and social care professions through life-long learning. A key aim of which is to reduce professional isolation, improve collaboration and the well-being of patients and their families.

Website: www.ihi.org/IHI/

INVOLVE

INVOLVE was established in 1996 and is part of, and funded by, the National Institute for Health Research, to support active public involvement in healthcare delivery and research. As a national advisory group, INVOLVE aims to bring together expertise, insight and experience in the field of public involvement, with the aim of advancing it as an essential part of the process by which research is identified, prioritised, designed, conducted and disseminated.

Website: www.invo.org.uk/

NORDIC INTERPROFESSIONAL NETWORK (NIPNET)

NIPNET is a learning network to foster interprofessional collaboration in education, practice and research. It is primarily for Nordic educators, practitioners and researchers in the fields of health. NIPNET is committed to interprofessional collaboration as a working model in healthcare and health and social services, with the intention to improve quality of care and health outcomes; and interprofessional education as learning models to develop interprofessional collaborative competences among health and social care services.

Website: www.nipnet.org/

PATIENT SAFETY NETWORK

(PSNet) is an initiative supported by the US Agency for Healthcare Research and Quality. It is a national web-based resource featuring the latest news and essential resources on patient safety. The site offers weekly updates of patient safety and teamwork literature, news, tools, and meetings, and a set of links to important research and other information on patient safety and team training and teamwork.

Website: www.psnet.ahrq.gov/

APPENDIX 12

Further reading

....

Below is a selection of further reading linked to collaboration among critical care professionals, and between patients/family members. We have presented these references in three main sections: general interprofessional reading; readings related to the themes presented in Chapter 2; and research/evaluation readings.

GENERAL READING

Balas, M.C., Burke, W.J., Gannon, D., Cohen, M.Z., Colburn, L., Ely, W. & Vasilevskis, E.E. (2013) Implementing the awakening and breathing coordination, delirium monitoring/management, and early exercise/mobility bundle into everyday care: Opportunities, challenges, and lessons learned for implementing the ICU pain, agitation, and delirium guidelines. *Critical Care Medicine*; 41(S9): 116–127.

Clay, A.S., Chudgar, S.M., Turner, K.M., Vaughn, J., Knudsen, N.W., Farnan, J.M., Arora, V.M., & Molloy, M.A. (2017) How prepared are medical and nursing students to identify common hazards in the intensive care unit? *Annals of the American Thoracic Society*; 14(4):543–549. DOI:10.1513/AnnalsATS.201610-773OC

Epstein, N.E. (2014) Multidisciplinary in-hospital teams improve patient outcomes: A review. *Surgical Neurology International*; 5(S7):295–303. DOI:10.4103/2152 7806.139612

Guidet, B. & González-Romá, V. (2011) Climate and cultural aspects in intensive care units. *Critical Care*; 15(6):312. DOI:http://ccforum.com/content/15/6/312

Guidet, B., van der Voort, P.H.J., & Csomos, A. (2017) Intensive care in 2050: Healthcare expenditure. *Intensive Care Medicine*; 43(8):1141–1143. DOI:10.1007/s00134-017-4679-2

Halpern, N.A. & Pastores, S.M. (2010) Critical care medicine in the United States 2000–2005: An analysis of bed numbers, occupancy rates, payer mix, and costs. *Critical Care Medicine*; 38(1):65–71. DOI:10.1097/CCM.0b013e3181b090d0

Holodinsky, J.K., Hebert, M.A., Zygun, D.A., Rigal, R., Berthelot, S., Cook, D.J. & Stelfox, H.T. (2015) A survey of rounding practices in Canadian adult intensive care units. *PLoS ONE*; 10(12):1–17. DOI:10.1371/journal.pone.0145408.

Jordan, J., Rose, L., Dainty, K.N., Noyes, J., & Blackwood, B. (2016) Factors that impact on the use of mechanical ventilation weaning protocols in critically ill adults and children: A qualitative evidence-synthesis. *Cochrane Database of Systematic Reviews*; 10. Art. No.: CD011812. DOI:10.1002/14651858.CD011812.pub2

Kvande, M., Lykkeslet, E. and Storli, S.L. (2017) ICU nurses and physicians dialogue regarding patients clinical status and care options: A focus group study, *International Journal of Qualitative Studies on Health and Well-being*; 12:1. DOI:10.1080/17482631.2016.1267346.

Kvarnstrom, S. (2008) Difficulties in collaboration: A critical incident study of inter-professional healthcare teamwork. *Journal of Interprofessional Care*; 22(2):191–203.

Lemieux-Charles, L. & McGuire, W.L. (2006) What do we know about health care team effectiveness? A review of the literature. *Medical Care Research and Review*; 63(3):263–300. DOI:10.1177/1077558706287003.

Neily, J., Mills, P.D., & Young-Xu, Y. (2010) Association between implementation of a medical team training program and surgical mortality. *JAMA*; 304(15):1693–1700.

Reader, T.W., Flin, R., Mearns, K. & Cuthbertson, B.H. (2007) Interdisciplinary communication in the intensive care unit. *British Journal of Anaesthesia*; 98(3): 347–352. DOI:10.1093/bja/ael372

Reader, T.W., Flin, R., Mearns, K., & Cuthbertson, B.H. (2009) Developing a team performance framework for the intensive care unit. *Critical Care Medicine*; 37(5): 1787–1793. DOI:10.1097/CCM.0b013e31819f0451

Rhodes, A., Moreno, R.P., Azoulay, E., Capuzzo, M., Chiche, J.D., Eddleston, J., Endacott, R., Ferdinande, P., Flaatten, H., Guidet, B., Kuhlen, R., Leo n-Gil, C., Martin Delgado, M.C., Metnitz, P.G., Soares, M., Sprung, C.L., Timsit, J.F., & Valentin, A. (2012) Prospectively defined indicators to improve the safety and quality of care for critically ill patients: A report from the Task Force on Safety and Quality of the European Society of Intensive Care Medicine. *Intensive Care Medicine*; 38:598–605. DOI:10.1007/s00134-011-2462-3.

Ridley, S. & Morris, S. (2007) Cost effectiveness of adult intensive care in the UK. *Anaesthesia*; 62:547–554. DOI:10.1111/j.1365-2044.2007.04997.x

Rodriquez, J. (2015) Who is on the medical team? Shifting the boundaries of belonging on the ICU. *Social Science & Medicine*; 144:112–118.

Seidel, J., Whiting, P.D., & Edbrooke, D.L. (2006) The costs of intensive care: Continuing education in anesthesia. *Critical Care & Pain*; 6(4):160–163. DOI:10.1093/bjaceaccp/mkl030.

Xyrichis, A., Lowton, K., Rafferty, A.M. (2017) Accomplishing professional jurisdiction in intensive care: An ethnographic study of three units. *Social Science & Medicine*; 181:102–111.

INTERPROFESSIONAL AND PATIENT/FAMILY COLLABORATION READING

Building the infrastructure to support sustainable improvement

Bongiovanni, T., Long, T., Khan, A.M., & Siegel, M.D. (2015) Bringing specialties together: The power of intra-professional teams. *Journal of Graduate Medical Education*; 7(1):19–20.

Weaver, S.J., Dy, S.M., Rosen, M.A. (2014) Team-training in healthcare: A narrative synthesis of the literature. *BMJ Quality and Safety*; 0:1–14. DOI:10.1136/bmjqs-2013-001848

Understanding how local context impacts collaboration

Barson, S., Doolan-Noble, F., Gray, J., & Gauld, R. (2017) Healthcare leaders' views on successful quality improvement initiatives and context. *Journal of Health Organization and Management*; 31(1):54–63. DOI:10.1108/JHOM-10-2016-0191.

Carrothers, K.M., Barr, J., Spurlock, B., Ridgely, M.S., Damberg, C.L., & Ely, W. (2013) Contextual issues influencing implementation and outcomes associated with integrated approach to managing pain, agitation, and delirium in adult ICUs. *Critical Care Medicine*; 41(S9):S128-S135. DOI:10.1097/CCM.0b013e3182a2c2b1.

Dixon-Woods, M., Leslie, M., Bion, J., & Tarrant, C. (2012) What counts? An ethnographic study of infection data reported to a patient safety program. *The Milbank Quarterly*; 90(3):548–591.

Gershengorn, H.B., Kocher, R., & Factor, P. (2014) Management strategies to effect change in intensive care units: Lessons from the world of business part I. Targeting quality improvement initiatives. *Annals of the American Thoracic Society*; 11(2):264–269. DOI:10.1513/AnnalsATS.201306-177AS.

Gershengorn, H.B., Kocher, R., & Factor, P. (2014) Management strategies to effect change in intensive care units: Lessons from the world of business part II. Quality-improvement strategies. *Annals of the American Thoracic Society*; 11(3):444–453. DOI:10.1513/AnnalsATS.201311-392AS.

Gershengorn, H.B., Kocher, R., & Factor, P. (2014) Management strategies to effect change in intensive care units: Lessons from the world of business part III. Effectively effecting and sustaining change. *Annals of the American Thoracic Society*; 11(3):454–457. DOI:10.1513/AnnalsATS.201311-393AS.

McDonald, K.M. (2013) Considering context in quality improvement interventions and implementation: Concepts, frameworks, and application. *Academic Pediatrics*; 13: S45–S53.

Øvretveit, J. (2011) Understanding the conditions for improvement: Research to discover which context influences affect improvement success. *BMJ Quality and Safety*; 20(S1):i18–i23. DOI:10.1136/bmjqs.2010.045955.

Stocker, M., Pilgrim, S.B., Burmester, M., Allen, M.L., & Gijselaers, W.H. (2016) Interprofessional team management in pediatric critical care: Some challenges and possible solutions, *Journal of Multidisciplinary Healthcare*; 9:47–58. DOI:http://dx.doi.org/10.2147/JMDH.S76773

The Matching Michigan Collaboration and Writing Committee (2012) Matching Michigan: A 2-year stepped interventional programme to minimize central venous catheter-blood stream infections in intensive care units in England. *BMJ Quality and Safety*; 1–14. DOI:10.1136/bmjqs-2012-001325.

van Dijk-de Vries, A., van Dongen, J.J., & van Bokhoven, M.A. (2017) Sustainable interprofessional teamwork needs a team-friendly healthcare system: Experiences from a collaborative Dutch programme. *Journal of Interprofessional Care*; 31(2):167–169. DOI:10.1080/13561820.2016.1237481.

CREATING PSYCHOLOGICALLY SAFE ENVIRONMENTS

Aranzamendez, G., James, D., & Toms, R. (2015) Finding antecedents of psychological safety: A step toward quality improvement. *Nursing Forum*; 50(3):171–178.

Edmondson, A. (1999) Psychological safety and learning behavior in work teams. *Administrative Science Quarterly*; 44(2):350–383.

Eppich, W. (2015) "Speaking Up" for Patient Safety in the Pediatric Emergency Department. *Clinical Pediatric Emergency Medicine*; 16(2):83–89.

Fagan, A., Parker, V., Jackson, D. (2016) A concept analysis of undergraduate nursing students speaking up for patient safety in the patient care environment. *Journal of Advanced Nursing*; 72(10):2346–2357. DOI:10.1111/jan.13028.

Fagan, M.J. (2012) Techniques to improve patient safety in hospitals: What nurse administrators need to know. *JONA*; 42(9):426–430. DOI:10.1097/NNA.0b013e3182664df5.

Frazier, M.L., Fainshmidt, S., Klinger, R.L., Pezeshkan, A., & Vracheva, V. (2016) Psychological safety: A meta-analytic review and extension. *Personnel Psychology*; 70:113–165. DOI:10.1111/peps.12183.

Maxfield, D., Grenny, J., Lanandero, R., Groah, L. (2011) *The silent treatment. Why safety tools and checklists aren't enough to save lives.* Available at: www.psqh.com/analysis/the-silent-treatment-why-safety-tools-and-checklists-arent-enough/

Newman, A., Donohue, R., & Eva, N. (2017). Psychological safety: A systematic review of the literature. *Human Resource Management Review*; 27(3):521–535. DOI:http://dx.doi.org/10.1016/j.hrmr.2017.01.001

O'Leary, D.F. (2016) Exploring the importance of team psychological safety in the development of two interprofessional teams. *Journal of Interprofessional Care*; 30(1):29–34. DOI:10.3109/13561820.2015.1072142

Tucker, A.L., Nembhard, I.M., & Edmondson, A.C. (2007) Implementing new practices: An empirical study of organizational learning in hospital intensive care units. *Management Science*; 53(6):894–907.

GIVING PATIENTS AND THEIR FAMILIES VOICE

Agard, A.S. & Maindal, H.T. (2009) Interacting with relatives in intensive care unit: Nurses' perceptions of a challenging task. *Nursing in Critical Care*; 14(5):264–272.

Back, A.L. & Arnold, R.M. (2013) "Isn't There Anything More You Can Do?": When empathic statements work, and when they don't. *Journal of Palliative Medicine*; 16(11):1429–1432. DOI:10.1089/jpm.2013.0193.

Bailey J.J., Sabbagh, M., Loiselle, C.G., Johanne Boileau, J., & McVey, L. (2010) Supporting families in the ICU: A descriptive correlational study of informational support, anxiety, and satisfaction with care. *Intensive and Critical Care Nursing*; 26:114–122.

Cypress, B.S. (2011) The lived ICU experience of nurses, patients and family members: A phenomenological study with Merleau-Pontian perspective. *Intensive and Critical Care Nursing*; 27:273–280. DOI:10.1016/j.iccn.2011.08.

Gro, F., Bjorg, D., Ashild, S. (2015) Family members' experiences of being cared for by nurses and physicians in Norwegian intensive care units: A phenomenological hermeneutical study. *Intensive and Critical Care Nursing*; 31:232–240. DOI:http://dx.doi.org/10.1016/j.iccn.2015.01.006

Haines, K.J., Kelly, P., Fitzgerald, P. Skinner, E.H, & Iwashyna, T.J (2017) The untapped potential of patient and family engagement in the organization of critical care. *Critical Care Medicine*; 45(5):899–906. DOI:10.1097/CCM.000000000000 2282.

Hupcey, J.E. (1999) Looking out for patient and ourselves – the process of family integration into the ICU. *Journal of Clinical Nursing*; 8:253–262.

Lane, D., Ferri, M., Lemaire, J., McLaughlin, K., & Stelfox, H.T. (2013) A systematic review of evidence-informed practices for patient care rounds in the ICU. *Critical Care Medicine*; 41(8):2016–2029. DOI:10.1097/CCM.0b013e31828a435f.

Lee Char, S.J., Evans, L.R., Malvar, G.L., & Douglas B. (2010) A randomized trial of two methods to disclose prognosis to surrogate decision makers in intensive care units. *American Journal of Respiratory Critical Care Medicine*; 182:905–909. DOI:10.1164/rccm.201002-0262OC.

Mitchell, M.L. & Chaboyerb, W. (2010) Family centred care – A way to connect patients, families and nurses in critical care: A qualitative study using telephone interviews. *Critical Care Nursing*; 26:154–160. DOI:10.1016/j.iccn.2010.03.003.

Schenker, Y., White, D.B., Crowley-Matoka, M., Dohan, D., Tiver, G.A., & Arnold, R.M. (2013) "It hurts to know. And it helps": Exploring how surrogates in the ICU cope with prognostic information. *Journal of Palliative Medicine*; 16(3): 243–249. DOI:10.1089/jpm.2012.0331.

Selph, R.B., Shiang, J., Engelberg, R., Curtis, R., White, D.B. (2008) Empathy and life support decisions in intensive care units. *Journal of General Internal Medicine*; 23(9):1311–1317. DOI:10.1007/s11606-008-0643-8.

Sevransky, J.E., Nicholl, B., Nicholl, J-B., & Buchman, T.G. (2017) Patient- and family-centered care: First steps on a long journey. *Critical Care Medicine*; 45(5):757–758. DOI:10.1097/CCM.0000000000002431.

Shaw, D.J., Davidson, J.E., Smilde, R.I., Sondoozi, T., & Agan, D. (2014) Multi-disciplinary team training to enhance family communication in the ICU. *Critical Care Medicine*; 42:265–271.

Söderströma, I.K., Saveman, B-I, Hagberg, M.S., & Benzein, E.G. (2009) Family adaptation in relation to a family member's stay in ICU. *Intensive and Critical Care Nursing*; 25:250–257. DOI:10.1016/j.iccn.2009.06.006.

van den Broek, J.M., Brunsveld-Reinders, A.H., Zedlitz, A.M., Girbes, A.R., de Jonge, E., & Arbous, M.S. (2015) Questionnaires on family satisfaction in the adult ICU: A systematic review including psychometric properties. *Critical Care Medicine*; 43:1731–1744.

Warrillow, S., Farley, K.J., & Jones, D. (2015) Ten practical strategies for effective communication with relatives of ICU patients. *Intensive Care Medicine*; 41: 2173–2176. DOI:10.1007/s00134-015-3815-0.

Zier, L.S., Burack, J.H., Micco, G., Chipman, A.K., Frank, J.A., White, D.B. (2012) Surrogate decision makers' interpretation of prognostic information: A mixed-methods study. *Annals of Internal Medicine*; 156:360–366.

INTERPROFESSIONAL EDUCATION

Barr, H., Gray, R., Helme, M. Low, H. & Reeves, S. (2016) *Interprofessional Education Guidelines*. CAIPE. Available at: www.caipe.org/resources/publications/

caipe-publications/barr-h-gray-r-helme-m-low-h-reeves-s-2016-interprofessional-education-guidelines

Barr, H., Koppel, I., Reeves, S., Hammick, M., & Freeth, D. (2005) *Effective Interprofessional Education: Assumption, Argument and Evidence*. London: Blackwell.

Delisle, M., Grymonpre, R., Whitley, R, Wirtzfeld, D. (2016) Crucial conversations: An interprofessional learning opportunity for senior healthcare students. *Journal of Interprofessional Care*; 30(6):777–786. DOI:10.1080/13561820.2016.1215971

Ericson, A., Lofgren, S., Bolinder, G., Reeves, S., Kitto, S., & Masiello, I. (2017) Interprofessional education in a student-led emergency department: A realist evaluation. *Journal of Interprofessional Care*; 31(2):199–206. DOI:10.1080/1356 1820.2016.1250726.

Freeth, D., Hammick, M., Reeves, S., Koppel, I., & Barr, H. (2005) *Effective Interprofessional Education: Development, Delivery and Evaluation*. London: Blackwell.

Hammick, M., Olckers, L., & Campion-Smith, C. (2009) Learning in interprofessional teams: AMEE Guide No 38. *Medical Teacher*; 31:1–12. DOI:10.1080/01421590 802585561.

Mitzkat, A., Berger, S., Reeves, S., & Mahler, C. (2016) More terminological clarity in the interprofessional field – a call for reflection on the use of terminologies, in both practice and research, on a national and international level. *GMS Journal of Medical Education*; 33(2). Doc36

Reeves, S., Palaganas, J., & Zierler, B. (2017) An updated synthesis of review evidence of interprofessional education. *Journal of Allied Health*; 46:56–61.

RESEARCH AND EVALUATION

Bernard, R. (2002) *Research Methods in Anthropology: Qualitative and Quantitative Approaches*. Walnut Creek, CA: AltaMira Press.

Gomm, R., Needham, G. & Bullman, A. (Eds) (2000). *Evaluating Research in Health and Social Care*. London: Sage.

Moustakas, C (1994) *Phenomenological research methods London*. Sage: London.

O'Brien, R. (2001*)* An Overview of the Methodological Approach of Action Research. In Richardson R (Ed.), *Theory and Practice of Action Research*. Available at: www.web.ca/~robrien/papers/arfinal.html

Ramsay, C., Matowe, L., Grilli, R., Grimshaw, J., Thomas, R. (2003) Interrupted time series designs in health technology assessment: Lessons from two systematic reviews of behavior change strategies. *International Journal of Technology Assessment in Health Care*; 19(4):613–623.

Reeves, S., Boet, S., Zierler, B., & Kitto, S. (2015) Interprofessional education and practice guide no. 3: Evaluating interprofessional education. *Journal of Interprofessional Care*; 29(4):305–312.

Rossi, P., Lipsey, M., & Freeman, H. (2004) *Evaluation: A Systematic Approach*. London: Sage.

Wludyka, P. (2011) Study designs and their outcomes. In: K. Macha & J. McDonough (Eds.), *Epidemiology for Advanced Nursing Practice*. Sudbury, MA: Jones and Bartlett Learning.

Glossary

Critical care – is specialised care delivered to patients whose conditions are life-threatening and who require comprehensive care and constant monitoring, usually in intensive care units (see below).

CUSP (Comprehensive Unit Based Safety Program) – is a five-step patient safety program designed to change workplace culture through education, organisational resources and interventions. (Also see Appendix 2.)

Ethnography – is a type of qualitative research that studies people in their everyday life through observing their behaviours and interactions and interviewing them. Ethnography in healthcare aims to shed light on issues between what professionals say they do and what they actually do in practice.

Formative evaluation – is usually undertaken during the development of interventions, programmes and initiatives. Its aim is to understand the nature of the early processes, outcomes and impact of activities in order to improve them.

Intensivist – is a physician who specialises in the care of critically ill patients, most often in the intensive care unit.

Intensive care unit (ICU) – are specialist hospital wards that provide treatment for patients who are critically ill. ICUs are staffed with specially-trained healthcare professionals.

Interprofessional collaboration (IPC) – occurs when different health and social care professions regularly come together to solve problems or provide services. Also referred to as *collaborative practice*.

Interprofessional communication – is the open and collaborative communication between health and social care professionals/students, and patients and families.

Interprofessional education – is a form of health professions education that involves members (or students) of two or more health and/or social care professions engage in learning with, from and about each other to improve collaboration and the delivery of care.

Interprofessional interventions – involve two or more health and social care professionals who learn and/or work together to improve their approach to collaboration.

Interprofessional teamwork – is a type of work which involves different health and/or social care professions who share a team identity and work closely together in an integrated and interdependent manner to solve problems and deliver services.

Patient/family involvement – is a highly subjective term that varies depending on the individual(s). Involvement is a complex and dynamic concept that not only includes the visible activities and interactions between people, but also the thoughts, feelings and meanings that people associate with these activities and interactions.

PROC framework – this framework was developed to help illuminate the complex array of factors that interprofessional teams may encounter in their daily practice. It includes four key domains: processual, relational, organisational and contextual factors (also see Reeves et al. 2010).

Quality improvement (QI) – is a collaborative intervention that consists of systematic and continuous actions that lead to measurable improvement in healthcare services and the health status of targeted patient groups.

Randomised control trial – is a test of the efficacy of an intervention which seeks to control for intervening variables by randomly allocating subjects into either an intervention group or a control group. It may be blind, double blind or triple blind depending on whether subjects, researchers or practitioners have knowledge of the group (intervention or control) to which a subject is allocated.

Safety culture – this term includes healthcare professionals' value systems and their patterns of clinical behaviour. For example, how healthcare professionals share physical space and team communication.

Summative evaluation – aims to judge the success of interventions, programmes and initiatives in relation to their "final" outcome(s) and impact. This type of evaluation is usually undertaken to account for resources and also to inform future planning.

Triangulation – is a technique which involves the comparison of findings from different methods (interviews, surveys), theories and/or perspectives of different people to generate more comprehensive insights.

Validity – refers to the degree to which a study or tool data collection (i.e. survey) accurately reflects the phenomena that the researcher is attempting to investigate/measure.

References

Agård, A.S., & Lomborg, K. (2011) Flexible family visitation in the intensive care unit: Nurses' decision-making. *Journal of Clinical Nursing*; 20(7–8):1106–1114. DOI:10.1111/j.1365-2702.2010.03360.x.

Agård, A.S., & Maindal, H.T. (2009) Interacting with relatives in intensive care unit: Nurses' perceptions of a challenging task. *Nursing in Critical Care*; 4(5):264–272. DOI:10.1111/j.1478-5153.2009.00347.x.

Appellebaum, N.P., Dow, A., Mazmanian, P.E., Jundt, D.K., & Applebaum, E.N. (2016) The effects of power, leadership and psychological safety on resident event reporting. *Medical Education*; 50:343–350. DOI:10.1111/medu.12947.

Austin, J.M. & Pronovost, P.J. (2015) "Never Events" and the quest to reduce preventable harm. *The Joint Commission Journal on Quality and Patient Safety*; 41(6):279–288.

Barr H., Hammick, M., Koppel, I., & Reeves, S. (1999) Evaluating interprofessional education: Two systematic reviews for health and social care. *British Education Research Journal*; 25(4):533–544.

Barr, H., Koppel, I., Reeves, S., Hammick, M., & Freeth, D. (2005) *Effective Interprofessional Education: Argument, Assumption, and Evidence*. Oxford and Malden, PA: Blackwell.

Bion, J., Richardson, A., Hibbert, P., Beer, J., Abrusci, T., McCutcheon, M., Cassidy, J., Eddleston, J., Gunning, K., Bellingan, G., Patten, M., & Harrison D. (2012) "Matching Michigan": A 2-year stepped interventional programme to minimise central venous catheter-blood stream infections in intensive care units in England. *BMJ Quality and Safety*; 22(2); 110–123.

Black, P., Boore, J., & Parahoo, K. (2011) The effect of nurse-facilitated family participation in the psychological care of the critically ill patient. *Journal of Advanced Nursing*; 67(5):1091–1101.

Blanchard, D., & Alavi, C. (2008). Asymmetry in the intensive care unit: Redressing imbalance and meeting the needs of family. *Nursing in Critical Care*; 13(5): 225–231.

Blom, H., Gustavsson, C., Johansson Sundler, A. (2013) Participation and support in intensive care as experienced by close relatives of patients – A phenomenological study. *Intensive & Critical Care Nursing*; 29:1–8.

Broyles, L.M., Tate, J.A., Happ Beth, M. (2012) Use of augmentative and alternative communication strategies by family members in the intensive care unit. *American Journal of Critical Care*; 21(2):e21–32. DOI:10.4037/ajcc2012752.

Burdick, K., Kara, A., Ebright, P., & Meek, J. (2017) Bedside interprofessional rounding: The view from the patient's side of the bed. *Journal of Patient Experience*; 4(1):22–27.

Burns, N. & Grove, S. (2009) *The Practice of Nursing Research: Appraisal, Synthesis, and Generation of Evidence.* (6th ed). St. Louis, MO: Saunders Elsevier.

Caldwell, D.F., Chatman, J., O'Reilly III, C.A., Ormiston, M., & Lapiz, M. (2008) Implementing strategic change in a health care system: The importance of leadership and change readiness. *Health Care Management Reviews*; 33(2):124–133.

Centers for Disease Control and Prevention. (2016) Healthcare-associated infections. Available at: www.cdc.gov/hai/surveillance/

Checkley, W., Martin, G.S., Brown, S.M., Chang, S., Dabbagh, O., Fremont, R.D., Girard, T.D., Rice,T.W., Howell,M.D., Johnson, S.B., O'Brien, J., Park, P.K., Pastores, S.M., Patil, N.T., Pietropaoli, A.P., Putman, M., Rotello, L., Siner, J., Sajid, S., Murphy, D.J., Sevransky, J.E., & USCIITG-CIOS Investigators. (2014) Structure, process and annual intensive care unit mortality across 69 centers: United States Critical Illness and Injury Trials Group Critical Illness Outcomes Study (USCIITG-CIOS). *Critical Care Medicine*; 42(2):344–356. DOI:10.1097/CCM.0b013e3182a275d7.

Chiang, C.L.V. (2011) Surviving a critical illness through mutually being there with each other: A grounded theory study. *Intensive & Critical Care Nursing*; 27:317–330.

Clevenger, K. (2007) Improve staff satisfaction with team building retreats. *Nursing Management*; 38:22–24.

Coar, L. & Sim, J. (2006) Interviewing one's peers: Methodological issues in a study of health professionals. Scand. *Journal of Primary Health Care*; 24(4):251–256. DOI:10.1080/02813430601008479.

Costa, D.K., Barg, F.K., Asch, D.A., & Kahn, J.M. (2014) Facilitators of an interprofessional approach to care in medical and mixed medical/surgical ICUs: A multicenter qualitative study. *Research in Nursing and Health*; 37(4):326–335. DOI:10.1002/nur.21607.

Costa, D.K., Wallace, D.J., Kahn, J.M. (2015) The association between daytime intensivist physician staffing and mortality in the context of other ICU organizational practices: A multicenter cohort study. *Critical Care Medicine*; 43(11):275–282.

Courtenay, M., Nancarrow, S., & Dawson, D. (2013) Interprofessional teamwork in the trauma setting: A scoping review. *Human Resources for Health*; 11:57. DOI:https://doi.org/10.1186/1478-4491-11-57

Curtis, J.R., Treece, P.D., Nielsen, E.L., Gold, J., Ciechanowsk, P.S., Shannon, S.E., Khandelwal, N., Young, J.P., & Engelberg, R.A. (2016) Randomized trial of communication facilitators to reduce family distress and intensity of end-of-life care. *American Journal of Respiratory Critical Care Medicine*; 193(2):154–162.

Cypress, B.S. (2012) Family presence on rounds: A systematic review of literature. *Dimensions of Critical Care Nursing*; 31(1):53–64.

Davidson, J.E. (2013) Family presence on rounds in neonatal, pediatric and adult intensive care units. *Annals of the American Thoracic Society*; 10(2):152–156.

Davidson, J.E., Aslakson, R.A., Long, A.C., Puntillo, K.A., Kross, E.K., Hart, J., Cox, C.E., ... & Curtis, R. (2017) Guidelines for family-centered care in the neonatal, pediatric, and adult ICU. *Critical Care Medicine*; 45(1):104–128. DOI:10.1097/CCM.0000000000002169.

Davidson, J.E., Jones, C. & Bienvenu, O.J. (2012) Family response to critical illness: Postintensive care syndrome–family. *Critical Care Medicine*; 40(2):618–624. DOI:10.1097/CCM.0b013e318236ebf9.

Dietz, A.S., Pronovost, P.J., Mendez-Tellez, P.A., Wyskiel, R., Masteller, J.A., Thompson, D.A., & Rosen, M.A. (2014) A systematic review of teamwork in the intensive care unit: What do we know about teamwork, team tasks, and improvement strategies? *Journal of Critical Care*; 29:904–914.

Di Gangi, S., Naretto, G., Cravero, N., & Livigni, S. (2013) A narrative-based study on communication by family members in intensive care unit. *Journal of Critical Care*; 28(4):483–489.

Dixon-Woods, M., Bosk, C.L., Aveling, E.L., Goeschel, C.A., & Pronovost, P.J. (2011) Explaining Michigan: Developing an ex post theory of a quality improvement program. *The Milbank Quarterly*; 89(2):167–205.

Dixon-Woods, M., Myles, L., Tarrant, C., & Bion, J. (2013) Explaining matching Michigan: An ethnographic study of a patient safety program. *Implementation Science*; 8:70.

Edmondson, A. (1999) Psychological safety and learning behavior in work teams. *Administrative Science Quarterly*; 44(2):350–383.

Edmondson, A. & Lei, Z. (2014) Psychological safety: The history, renaissance, and future of an interpersonal construct. *Annual Review of Organizational and Psychological Behaviour*; 1:23–43. DOI:10.1146/annurev-orgpsych-031413-091305.

Egerod, I. & Bagger, C. (2010). Patients' experiences of intensive care diaries: A focus group study. *Intensive and Critical Care Nursing*; 26:278–287.

Fanelli, S. & Zangrandi, A. (2017) Assessment for improving performance of NICUs: The Italian experience. *Health Services Management Research*; 30(3):168–178.

Fox, A. & Reeves, S. (2015) Interprofessional collaborative patient-centred care: A critical exploration of two related discourses. *Journal of Interprofessional Care*; 29:113–118.

Fulbrook, P., Albarran, J.W., & Latour, J.M. (2005) A European survey of critical care nurses' attitudes and experiences of having family members present during cardiopulmonary resuscitation. *International Journal of Nursing Studies*; 42(5):557–568.

Gabelicaa, C., Van den Bosscheab, P., De Maeyerb, S., Segersa, M., Gijselaersa, W. (2014) The effect of team feedback and guided reflexivity on team performance change. *Learning and Instruction*; 34:86–96.

Gachoud, D., Albert, M., Kuper, A., Stroud, L., & Reeves, S. (2012) Meanings and perceptions of patient-centredness in social work, nursing and medicine: A comparative study. *Journal of Interprofessional Care*; 26:484–490.

Gerritsen, R.T., Hartog, C.S., & Curtis, J.R. (2017) New developments in the provision of family-centered care in the intensive care unit. *Intensive Care Medicine*; 43:550–553. DOI:10.1007/s00134-017-4684-5.

Halcomb, E.J. & Davidson, P.M. (2006) Is verbatim transcription of interview data always necessary? *Applied Nursing Research*; 19:38–42. DOI:10.1016/j.apnr.2005.06.001.

Halpern, N.A. & Pastores, S.M. (2015) Critical care medicine beds, use, occupancy, and costs in the United States: A methodological review. *Critical Care Medicine*; 43(11):2452–2459. DOI:10.1097/CCM.0000000000001227.

Happ, M. (2000) Interpretation of nonvocal behavior and the meaning of voicelessness in critical care. *Social Science and Medicine*; 50:1247–1255.

Hills, J. (2003) Organizing a practice retreat. *Journal of Medical Practice Management*; 19:97–99.

Institute of Medicine. (2000) *To err is human. Building a safer health system.* Washington, DC: National Academies Press.

Interprofessional Education Collaborative. (2016) *Core competencies for interprofessional collaborative practice: 2016 update.* Washington, DC: Interprofessional Education Collaborative.

Interprofessional Education Collaborative Expert Panel. (2011) *Core competencies for interprofessional collaborative practice. Report of an expert panel.* Washington, DC: Interprofessional Education Collaborative.

Johnson, C. (2009) Bad blood: Doctor-nurse behavior problems impact patient care. Available at: www.ache.org/policy/doctornursebehavior.pdf

Kahn, J.M. & Rubenfeld, G.D. (2015) The myth of the workforce crisis why the United States does not need more intensivist physicians. *American Journal of Respiratory and Critical Care Medicine*; 191(2):128–134. DOI:10.1164/rccm.201408-1477CP.

Kaplan, H.C., Froehle, C.M., Cassedy, A. Provost, L.P., Margolis, P.A. (2013) An exploratory analysis of the model for understanding success in quality. *Health Care Management Reviews*; 38(4):325–338. DOI:10.1097/HMR.0b013e3182689772.

Kaplan, H.C., Provost, L.P., Froehle, C.M., & Margolis, P.A. (2011) The model for understanding success in quality (MUSIQ): Building a theory of context in healthcare quality improvement. *BMJ Quality and Safety*; 21:13e20. DOI:10.1136/bmjqs-2011-000010.

Kean, S. & Mitchell, M. (2013) How do intensive care nurses perceive families in intensive care? Insights from the United Kingdom and Australia. *Journal of Clinical Nursing*; 23(5–6):663–72. DOI:10.1111/jocn.12195.

Kendall-Gallagher, D., Reeves, S., Alexanian, J., & Kitto, S. (2016) A nursing perspective of interprofessional work in critical care: A secondary analysis. *Journal of Critical Care*; 38:20–26.

Kerlin, M.P. Neill K. J. Adhikari, N.K., Rose, L., Wilcox, M.E., Bellamy, C.J., Costa, D.K., Gershengorn, H.B., Halpern, S.D., Kahn, J.M., Lane-Fall, M.B., Wallace, D.J., Weiss, C.H., Wunsch, H. and Cooke, C.R., on behalf of the ATS Ad Hoc Committee on ICU Organization. (2017) An official American Thoracic Society systematic review: The effect of nighttime intensivist staffing on mortality and length of stay among intensive care unit patients. *American Journal of Respiratory Critical Care Medicine*, 195(3):383–393. DOI:10.1164/rccm.201611-2250ST.

Kim, M.M., Barnato, A.E., Angus, D.C., Fleisher, L.F., & Kahn, J.M. (2010) The effect of multidisciplinary care teams on intensive care unit mortality. *Archives of Internal Medicine*; 170(4):369–376. DOI:10.1001/archinternmed.2009.521.

Kirkpatrick, D.L. (1967) Evaluation of training. In R. Crail & L. Bittel (Eds) *Training and Development Handbook.* New York: McGraw-Hill.

Konradt, U., Otte, K.P., Schippers, M.C., & Steenfatt, C. (2016) Reflexivity in teams: A review and new perspectives. *The Journal of Psychology*; 150:153–174.

Kringos, D.S., Sunol, R., Wagner, C., Mannion, R., Michel, P., Klazinga, N.S., & Groene, O. on behalf of the DUQuE Consortium (2015) The influence of context on the effectiveness of hospital quality improvement strategies: A review of systematic reviews. *BMC Health Services Research*; 15:277–278. DOI:10.1186/s12913-015-0906-0.

Leclair, L., Dawson, M., Howe, A., Hale, S., Zelman, E., Clouser, R., Garrison, G., & Allen, G. (2017) A longitudinal interprofessional simulation curriculum for critical care teams: Exploring successes and challenges. *Journal of Interprofessional Care*; DOI:10.1080/13561820.2017.1405920.

Lutfiyya, M.N., Brandt, B.F. & Cerra, F. (2016b) Reflections from the intersection of health professions education and clinical practice: The state of the science of interprofessional education and collaborative practice. *Academic Medicine*; 91:766–771.

Lutfiyya, M.N., Brandt, B.F., Delaney, C., Pechacek, J., & Cerra, F. (2016a) Setting a research agenda for interprofessional education and collaborative practice in the context of United States health system reform. *Journal of Interprofessional Care*; 30(1):7–14.

Manthous C & Hollingshead A. (2011) Team science and critical care. *American Journal of Respiratory Critical Care*; 184:17–25.

Manthous, C., Nembhard, I., & Hollingshead, A. (2011) Building effective critical care teams. *Critical Care*; 15(4):307. DOI:10.1186/cc10255.

McConnell, B. & Moroney, T. (2015) Involving relatives in ICU patient care: Critical care nursing challenges. *Journal of Clinical Nursing*; 24(7–8):991–998.

Miles M. & Huberman A. (1994) *Qualitative Data Analysis: An Expanded Sourcebook*. Thousand Oaks, CA: Sage.

Mischo-Kelling, M., Wieser, H., Cavada, L., Lochner, L., Vittadello, F., Fink, V., & Reeves, S. (2015) The state of interprofessional collaboration in Northern Italy: A mixed methods study. *Journal of Interprofessional Care*; 29;79–81.

Mitchell, M. & Chaboyer, W. (2010) Family-Centred Care-A way to connect patients, families and nurses in critical care: A qualitative study using telephone interviews. *Intensive and Critical Care Nursing*; 26(3):154–160. DOI:10.1016/j.iccn.2010.03.003.

Nelms, T. & Eggenberger, S. (2010) The essence of the family critical illness experience and nurse family meetings. *Journal of Family Nursing*; 16:462–486.

Nembard, I.M. & Edmondson, A.C. (2006) Making it safe: The effects of leader inclusiveness and professional status on psychological safety and improvement efforts in health care teams. *Journal of Organizational Behavior*; 27:941–966. DOI:10.1002/job.413.

Olding, M., McMillan, S.E., Reeves, S., Schmitt, M.H., Puntillo, K., & Kitto, S. (2016) Patient and family involvement adult critical care and intensive care settings: A scoping review. *Health Expectations*; 19:1183–1202.

Olsen, K.D., Dysvik, E., & Sætre, B. (2009) The meaning of family members' presence during intensive care stay: A qualitative study. *Intensive and Critical Care Nursing*; 25(4):190–198. DOI:10.1016/j.iccn.2009.04.004.

Onwuegbuzie, A. & Dickinson, W. (2008) Mixed methods analysis and information visualization: Graphical display for effective communication of research results. *The Qualitative Report*; 13(2):204–225.

Organisation for Economic Co-operation and Development (2016) OECD Reviews of Health Care Quality: Raising Standards. Available at: http://dx.doi.org/10.1787/9789264239487-en

Øvretveit, J. (1997) Planning and managing teams. *Health and Social Care in the Community*; 5:269–276.

Paradis, E., Leslie, M., Puntillo, K., Gropper, M., Aboumatar, H.J., Kitto, S., & Reeves, S. (2014) Delivering interprofessional care in intensive care settings: Results from a scoping review of qualitative studies. *American Journal of Critical Care*; 23(3):230–238.

Pinho D, Parreira C, Queiroz E, Abbad G, Reeves S (2018) Investigating the nature of interprofessional collaboration in primary care across the Western Health Region of Brasília, Brazil: A study protocol. *Journal of Interprofessional Care*; 32:228–230.

Prin, M. & Wunsch, H. (2012) International comparisons of intensive care: Informing outcomes and improving standards. *Current Opinion in Critical Care*; 18(6): 700–706. DOI:10.1097/MCC.0b013e32835914d5.

Pronovost, P.J., Goeschel, C.A., Colantuoni, E., Watson, S., Lubomski, L.H., Berenholtz, S.M., Thompson, D.A., Sinopoli, D.J., Cosgrove, S., Sexton, B., Marsteller, J.A., Hyzy, R.C., Welsh, R., Posa, P., Schumacher, K., & Needham, D. (2010) Sustaining reductions in catheter related bloodstream infections in Michigan intensive care units: An observational study. *BMJ*; 340: c309.

Pronovost, P., Needham, D., Berenholtz, S., Sinopoli, D., Chu, H., Cosgrove, S., Sexton, B., Hyzy, R., Welsh, R., Roth, G., Bander, J., Kepros, J., & Goeschel, C. (2006) An intervention to decrease catheter-related bloodstream infections in the ICU. *New England Journal of Medicine*; 355:2725–2732.

Reeves, S., Boet, S., Zierler, B., & Kitto, S. (2015b) Interprofessional education and practice guide No. 3: Evaluating interprofessional education. *Journal of Interprofessional Care*; 29(4):305–312.

Reeves, S., Clark, E., Lawton, S., Ream, M., & Ross, F. (2017b) Examining the nature of Interprofessional interventions designed to promote patient safety: a narrative review. *International Journal for Quality in Health Care*; 27:144–50.

Reeves, S., Fletcher, S., Barr, H., Birch, I., Boet, S., Davies, N., ... & Kitto, S. (2016). A BEME systematic review of the effects of interprofessional education: BEME Guide No. 39. *Medical Teacher*; 38:1–13. DOI:10.3109/0142159X.2016. 1173663.

Reeves, S. & Lewin, S. (2004) Hospital-based interprofessional collaboration: strategies and meanings. *Journal of Health Services Research and Policy*; 9:218–225.

Reeves, S., Lewin, S., Espin, S., & Zwarenstein, M. (2010) *Interprofessional Teamwork For Health And Social Care*. Oxford: Wiley-Blackwell.

Reeves S., McMillan S.E., Kachan N., Paradis E., Leslie M., & Kitto S. (2015a) Interprofessional collaboration and family member involvement in intensive care units: emerging themes from a multi-site ethnography. *Journal of Interprofessional Care*; 29(3):230–237.

Reeves, S., Pelone, F., Harrison, R., Goldman, J., & Zwarenstein, M. (2017a) Interprofessional collaboration: Effects of practice-based interventions on professional practice and healthcare outcomes (Update). *Cochrane Database of Systematic Reviews*. CD000072 DOI:10.1002/14651858.CD000072.pub3.

Reeves, S., Peller, J., Goldman, J., & Kitto, S. (2013) Ethnography in qualitative educational research: AMEE Guide No. 80. *Medical Teacher*; 8:e1365–1379.

Reeves, S., Rice, K., Gotlib Conn, L., Miller, K-L., Kenaszchuk, C., & Zwarenstein, M. (2009) Interprofessional interaction, negotiation and non-negotiation on general internal medicine wards. *Journal of Interprofessional Care*; 23:633–645.

Robert Wood Johnson Foundation (2015) Lessons from the field: Promising interprofessional practices. Available at: www.rwjf.org/en/library/research/2015/03/lessons-from-the-field.html

Robinson, C.A., & Wright, L.M. (1995) Family nursing interventions: What families say makes a difference. *Journal of Family Nursing*; 1:327–345.

Rosen, M.A., Salas, E., Wilson, K.A., King, H.B., Salisbury, M., Augenstein, J.S., Robinson, D.W., & Birnbach. D.J. (2008) Measuring team performance in simulation-based training: Adopting best practices for healthcare. *Simulation in Healthcare*; 3(1):33–41. DOI:10.1097/SIH.0b013e3181626276.

Salas, E., Diaz Granados, D., Klein, C., Burke, C.S., Stagl, K.C., Goodwin, G.F., & Halpin, S.M. (2008) Does team training improve team performance? A meta-analysis. *Human Factors*; 50:903–933.

Sharma, S., Boet, S., Kitto, S., & Reeves, S. (2011) Interprofessional simulated learning: The need for "sociological fidelity". *Journal of Interprofessional Care*; 25:81–83.

Shelton, W., Moore, C.D., Socaris, S., Gao, J., & Dowling, J. (2010) The effect of a family support intervention on family satisfaction, length-of-stay, and cost of care in the intensive care unit. *Critical Care Medicine*; 38(5):1315–1320.

Siedlecki, S. & Hixson, E. (2015) Relationships between nurses and physicians matter. *The Online Journal of Issues in Nursing*; 20(3). DOI:10.3912/OJIN.Vol20No03PPT03.

Söderström, I-M., Saveman, B-I., Hagberg, M.S., & Benzein, E.G. (2009) Family adaptation in relation to a family member's stay in ICU. *Intensive & Critical Care Nursing*; 25(5):250–257. DOI:10.1016/j.iccn.2009.06.006.

Sullivan, D.R., Liu, X., Corwin, D.S., Verceles, A.C., McCurdy, M.T., Pate, D.A., Davis, J.M., & Netzer, G. (2012) Learned helplessness among families and surrogate decision-makers of patients admitted to medical, surgical, and trauma ICUs. *Chest*; 142(6):1440–1446. DOI:10.1378/chest.12-0112.

Thomas, C.M., Bertram, E., & Johnson, S. (2009) The SBAR Communication Technique. *Nurse Educator*; 34 (4):176–180. DOI:10.1097/NNE.0b013e3181aaba54.

Valentin, A., Ferdinande, P. & ESICM Working Group on Quality Improvement (2011) Recommendations on basic requirements for intensive care units: Structural and organizational aspects. *Intensive Care Medicine*; 37(10):1575–1587. DOI:10.1007/s00134-011-2300-7.

Van Den Bos, J., Rustagi, K., Gray,T., Halford, M., Ziemkiewicz, E. & Shreve, J. (2011) The $17.1 billion problem: The annual cost of measurable medical error. *Health Affairs*; 30(4):596–603. DOI:10.1377/hlthaff.2011.0084.

Vico Chiang C.L (2011) Surviving a critical illness through mutually being there with each other: A grounded theory study. *Intensive & Critical Care Nursing*; 27(6): 317–330.

Vincent, J.L., Marshall, J.C., Ñamendys-Silva, S.A., FranÇois, B., Martin-Loeches, I., Lipman, J., Reinhart, K., Antonelli, M., Pickkers, P., Njimi, H., Jimenez, E., & Sakr, Y. (2014) Assessment of the worldwide burden of critical illness: The Intensive Care Over Nations (ICON) audit. *Lancet Respiratory Medicine*; 2:380–386.

Weled, B.J., Adzhigirey, L.A., Hodgman, T.M., Brilli, R.J., Spevetz, A., Kline, A.M., Montgomery, V.L., Puri, N., Tisherman, S.A., Vespa, P.M., Pronovost, P.J., Rainey,

T.G., Patterson, A.J., & Wheeler, D. (2015) Critical care delivery: The importance of process of care and ICU structure to improved outcomes: An update from the American college of critical medicine task force on models of critical care. *Critical Care Medicine*; 43(7):1520–1525.

West, M. (1996) *Handbook of Work Group Psychology*. Chichester, UK: Wiley.

Windsor, L.C. (2013) Using concept mapping in community-based participatory research: A mixed methods approach. *Journal of Mix Methods Research*; 7: 274–293.

Wright, L. M., & Leahey, M. (2009). *Nurses and Families: A Guide to Family Assessment and Intervention* (5th ed.). Philadelphia, PA: FA Davis.

Index

Page numbers in *italics* refer to figures. Page numbers in **bold** refer to tables.